THE
Slim-Fast®
MAKEOVER

THE Slim·Fast®

MAKEOVER

14 DAY PLAN TO KICK-START WEIGHT LOSS AND CHANGE YOUR LIFESTYLE

LAUREN HUTTON

WITH DEBORAH KOTZ

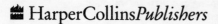 HarperCollins*Publishers*

HarperCollins*Publishers*
77–85 Fulham Palace Road,
Hammersmith, London W6 8JB

HarperCollins website address is: www.**fire**and**water**.com
Slim•Fast™ website address is: www.slim-fast.com

First published in the USA by ReganBooks 2000
This edition published by HarperCollins 2000

1 3 5 7 9 10 8 6 4 2

© The Slim•Fast Foods Company 2000

The Slim•Fast Foods Company asserts the moral right to be
identified as the author of this work

A catalogue record of this book is
available from the British Library

ISBN 0 00 710955 5

Printed and bound in Great Britain by
Omnia Books Ltd, Glasgow

contents

This book contains information relating to losing weight and weight maintenance. It is not intended to replace medical advice. Rather, the information provided should be used to supplement regular care by medical professionals. Several particular warnings are in order: if you want to lose weight and are under 18, pregnant, nursing, following a diet recommended by a doctor, have health problems, or want to lose more than 30lbs, see a doctor before starting the Slim•Fast programme or any other weight loss programme. No-one should lose more than 2lbs per week after the first week on a weight loss programme. Rapid weight loss may cause health problems.

This book follows the American dietary recommendations, followed by the Slim•Fast Foods Company. You will find that the eating programme in this book recommends a higher number of calories than the recommendations in the Slim•Fast booklet in the UK, which follows the EU Directive on slimming products.

Very occasionally, where the editor for this UK edition has had to adapt a recipe where a certain American-produced ingredient was not available in this territory, it may not have been possible to alter the Nutritional Information Per Serving. The variation, in such cases, will only be very minor.

Slim•Fast and I

Even when I was just beginning my career in the mid-1960s, I could-n't model anything I didn't believe in. On the very first Paris collection I ever shot for Vogue magazine, I was handed a leopard-skin coat – and handed it right back. I just couldn't put it on. It almost made me cry. This could easily have been the end of my career; you don't say no to Vogue when things are just getting started for you. I told the editor why I couldn't wear the coat and why I didn't think they should show it; she told the photographer; somebody called Diana Vreeland, Vogue's poohbah, and not only did they drop the leopard coats (instead of me!) from their pages that year, but Vreeland also dropped a word at a Washington dinner soon there-after, and the next thing you know, it was illegal to import wild spotted fur into America.

So I learned early on about influence. The day the surgeon general announced that smoking was harmful to one's health, I saw Irving Penn talking on the phone to his agent and forbidding him to take any cigarette accounts – giving up some serious money. A little while later a cigarette company asked me to do a giant campaign for them, offering more money than I'd ever been offered for a job until that time. I was still a smoker myself, but I said absolutely not – I may have been a user (back then), but I wasn't a pusher. I've always tried to take care with the associations I make, so I'll never have to look back later and wonder whether I may have harmed anyone.

When I first started hearing about Slim•Fast, I was sceptical. I'd spent my last thirty-six professional years as Ms. Natural. For ages I've tried to be careful about what I ate, and a lot of my family and friends are health-food devotees or vegetarians. One of my sisters has been organic-only since the 1960s, and her children have never even had anything cooked in animal or fish stock, much less actually eaten any meat. Serious vegans forever. 'You are what you eat' was one of the youthful slogans of my slogan-happy generation.

But the truth is that in recent years I hadn't been feeling as good about my body as I used to – and for good reason. Over a period of fifteen years, I'd put on 22 per cent of my original body weight – going from 115 to 140 pounds. When I realized that, I knew I had to make a change in my lifestyle. When I was home I'd eat right, but too often I found myself on the run, eating my way through room-service menus at the nicer hotels or grabbing fast food when I was pushed for time. I've done a lot of movies and when you're on a location shoot you often spend ten hours a day waiting and only a few working; when you're waiting that long, one of the few things you have to look forward to is food, and sometimes I'd order more than I should, just hoping I'd find something that tasted good.

After all, I was young and as slim as I'd ever be; I didn't have to watch my weight … or so I thought, until I woke up one day 25 pounds heavier than I'd ever been. Once I turned forty, my body no longer felt the way it always had; all at once it felt uncomfortable, like a heavy, ill-fitting suit of clothes. I'd never felt my thighs rubbing together, but there they were! Suddenly my upper arms were brushing against my sides – at first I didn't even know what that feeling was. At work I started standing sideways to look thinner – it was amazing that I managed to fake my way through modelling as long as I did.

And it wasn't just the weight that bothered me; I just didn't have the energy I used to. At around this time I also attended a medical programme to help me quit smoking, which taught me a lot about health but left me more concerned than ever about the state of my body. I tried for years to take off the weight, but I hated the idea of a diet – I couldn't even stand to use the word. But I knew I had to do something.

That's when I first started thinking about trying a programme like Slim●Fast. Of course, not everyone had an open mind when I broached the subject with them. Many of my friends – including the ones who'd known me the longest – couldn't believe what I was saying. But Slim●Fast comes in a can!, they said. And I have to admit that I had my doubts, too. It sounded like the kind of quick-fix gimmick my generation had always been taught to resist.

But then something happened that really got my attention, and it involved one of my favourite things to do in life – scuba diving.

Ever since one brilliant day in Cozumel, Mexico, in 1965, when I first walked into the sea wearing a scuba tank, I've been a fanatic about diving. For about fifteen years after that I dived all over the world, whenever I had the chance, until my once-stable personal life began getting the bends and scuba diving became less of a priority. But in recent years I'd really begun to miss it, and in 1997 I finally got started again when I headed for the wreck diver's Valhalla – the Truk Lagoon in Micronesia, where during World War II American bombers sunk more than forty Japanese munitions boats and shot down more than thirty Zero fighter planes. Half a century later they're still there, 60–180 feet below the surface; covered in masses of soft coral in bright red, orange and yellow, they look like the product of a summit meeting between Michelangelo and Walt Disney. The diving there is unbeatable, and my love affair with diving was rekindled immediately.

Diving is exhilarating; taking the plunge into that lagoon is like falling backward into Botticelli's clamshell, arms outstretched – Venus laughing. But it's also tough business. When you're scurrying around more than a hundred feet below the surface, you're often subject to vicious currents – and when a thick wave of silt is stirred up in the atmosphere around you, it can be difficult to find the way out. That's why I was so glad to meet my true dive buddies when I started diving seriously again – a bunch of world-class divers who make a living out of all this adventure. Mitch Scaggs, Tanya Burnett, Brett Gillum and Dan Ruth: these are the bad boys (and girl) who allow me to join their underwater team whenever I'm in their neck of the woods – which is anywhere in the world.

Whenever I get a new idea, I have a habit of polling my closest friends, the ones who know me best, to see whether they think it makes sense. So when I began thinking about trying Slim•Fast, I mentioned it to my diving pals. I didn't know what to expect; this is a pretty macho bunch, after all. But I sure didn't expect the response I got: they'd all used Slim•Fast themselves, and they loved it. Dan had lost 50 pounds on it and he returns to it whenever his wetsuit gets a little tight. These professional divers are some pretty tough characters; they face danger every day and come up laughing. If they were Slim•Fast regulars, that told me one thing – those shakes obviously aren't for sissies.

So I started looking into Slim•Fast a little more deeply. I knew that what I needed was a way to get a calorie-controlled, nutritionally balanced diet every day, and I knew myself well enough to know that following it had better be easy. And what I learned is that the Slim•Fast Plan is no gimmick. It's a programme, designed by leading nutritionists and proven in decades of studies and consumer success stories, that helps you to achieve a balanced diet every day – to get your full complement of vitamins and nutrients, all wrapped up in two shakes a day and a sensible dinner. There's even an allowance for snacks on the side. With up to twenty-four vitamins and minerals going for it, it's a much healthier regime than most of us consume every day – certainly better than I was eating. And so I decided to try it.

The results? I loved the taste of the chocolate shake immediately; it tasted like the chocolate milk of my childhood. So I knew I could make Slim•Fast part of my life. There were no schedules to follow, no elaborate meals to prepare. It was versatile; if I knew I had to have a big business lunch, I could have a shake for breakfast and another one for dinner – and that in turn gave me more time to do other things, like sneaking in a little exercise or doing some reading.

And here's a thing you should know: it didn't all happen at once. Nothing's perfect in this world, and when I started off with Slim•Fast I didn't fully commit right away – I'd have a shake here and there but then get distracted by some appealing meal and fall off. But after a week or two I found myself sticking to the programme full-time – two shakes a day, a sensible meal and some moderate exercise. And the most important thing was the simplest: it worked. I began losing weight, and feeling wonderful and energetic at the same time. By the time three weeks had passed I'd lost 7 pounds; a few weeks later I was down 12. At the age of fifty-six, I weighed 129 pounds for the first time since I was … thirty-six? Forty-one? I can't even remember. And I'm still losing! Recently I tried on a sleek red dress I've had for years – a real beauty that hasn't fitted me in ages – and it slipped right on! There's no other way to put it: I feel terrific.

And that's why I was happy about doing this book. The people at Slim•Fast have been helping folks lose weight and get healthy for decades; by now there are millions of us successful dieters using their shakes and bars on a regular basis. But the Slim•Fast team knows that staying healthy for life is about more than just dropping a few pounds – too many crash dieters have tried that quick-fix approach and then put the weight right back on as soon as they got tired of eating grapefruit or steak and eggs all day. When I first began meeting with Slim•Fast's medical experts, what really impressed me was their broader message: losing weight is a choice anyone can make. All it takes is a few minor adjustments in lifestyle: start eating right, find some exercises you enjoy, take a few steps to reduce stress in your life. And before you know it, the Slim•Fast Plan will have you looking better and feeling fantastic. We call it the Slim•Fast Makeover.

All Debbie Kotz and I have tried to do in this book is show you how to get your own makeover started. Along the way you'll hear from people like me who've been through just what you're going through now: remember, you can be one of the millions who are doing this successfully. Whether it's 7 pounds or 75 pounds you have to lose, all it takes is a little change in your eating habits, and they'll change before you know it. Once you're under way, I'll bet you'll find it as easy as I have to get fit and remake your life.

Get started! You'll be a new you before you know it. I know I am. And I'm rooting for you.

1

change your body, change your life

How many times have you stared at yourself in the mirror and thought, 'If only ...' If only I could be trimmer, fitter, healthier ... If only I could get into my old jeans ... Someday – maybe next September, next April, next summer, next year ... If only I could find a way to remake my life ...

When it comes to your body, you've probably spent a lot of time on this kind of wishful thinking. But the very fact that you're opening this book means you're ready to consider turning your 'if only's' into positive and lasting action.

Perhaps you've been overweight all your life, or perhaps, like many people, you've gone from fat to thin and back again. Or maybe you've only recently realized that the one or two pounds or kilograms you've been gaining every year have really added up.

Well, no matter what your circumstances, there's no time like the present to change your life. With the Slim•Fast Makeover, losing weight – and keeping it off for life – can be within your grasp. It's a plan that has been tested in universities and proven in households all over the world: through a combination of balanced nutrition, exercise and other beneficial changes in your way of living, you can have the body you want ... and the life you deserve.

If your weight is weighing heavily on your mind, you're certainly not alone. Losing weight is an obsession in our culture. Despite the fact that one in five people in Britain is obese, we're bombarded with images of impossibly slender actresses and models splashed across TV screens and the covers of countless magazines. What we don't see is their nonstop and often very unhealthy dieting.

In an effort to attain that kind of 'ideal' body, many of us have turned to sporadic dieting – only to be sorely disappointed in the end. For years, we've been searching in frustration for a quick-fix way to lose weight, in an attempt to trick our bodies into shedding those extra pounds. We earnestly believed that all-protein diets would keep us thin for life. Once we gained the weight back after going off those diets, we turned to the grapefruit diet, then the food-combining diet (eating certain foods at certain times of the day), and before we knew it we were back on the high-protein kick. But who wants to live under rigid eating rules for a lifetime? When the restrictions got too taxing, we dropped the diets and went back to our old eating habits.

No wonder we're fed up with trying to lose weight. Who can blame you if your first thought when hearing about a new weight-loss product or plan is: *What's the catch?*

Well, your instincts are right. Most such products and plans do have a catch: they're all temporary ways to take off weight, and none can ever promise that you'll stay thin forever. That's because when you buy into one of these gimmicks, you're buying into the notion that you're going on a diet just long enough to lose weight. Once you've lost the weight, you're led to believe that you can go AWOL and abandon any of the restrictions you were following.

You've probably heard this before, or experienced it firsthand: losing weight isn't the hardest part – it's keeping the pounds off that's tricky. Any yo-yo dieter can attest to this fact, and dieting statistics confirm it. As many as 75–90 per cent of people who lose weight eventually gain back the weight they've lost, and sometimes they gain even more.

The leading obesity experts now realize that most dieters haven't figured out what it takes to maintain weight loss – and that most weight-loss programmes don't really teach people to make the changes they'll need to keep the pounds off for life. Many such programmes focus on getting you to your goal weight without giving you the tools for staying there. The drastic behaviour changes most require to lose weight – from attending weekly sessions to restricting your diet to unpalatable foods – are usually too severe to stay on forever.

In order to beat the odds and be a successful dieter, you need to make small, simple changes that fit naturally into your lifestyle – this will allow you to lose the weight you want *and* keep it off for life.

This book is designed to help you do just that. The plan it offers, designed and refined by a team of nutritionists over more than two decades, can help you lose weight sensibly so you can live a long, healthy life. It will help you make over not only your body, but your mind and your life. And here's the best thing about it: simple and easy to follow, this plan can actually enable you to enjoy your life more than ever before. Once you start losing weight, you'll likely start feeling better, experience a greater sense of energy, have more self-confidence and exult in the knowledge that you've taken your health in your own hands.

The makeover is based on the proven Slim•Fast Plan that has helped countless dieters remake their bodies and transform their lives. Convenient, inexpensive, proven in years of medical trials, the Slim•Fast Plan has long been established as one of the healthiest and most dependable ways to lose weight.

Is Your Weight in the Danger Zone?

While you're weighing your decision about whether to embark on a journey to a new weight and a new life, you might want to consider the health implications of being overweight. You probably already know that obesity can lead to a host of health problems, from heart disease to diabetes. But how much is too much? If you're otherwise healthy, what's the harm in carrying an extra 18kgs (2 stones)? Plenty, according to the latest research. Being even moderately overweight carries certain health risks, and being obese is downright dangerous; one new study found that obese people have a two-and-a-half-times-greater chance of dying from weight-related illnesses than those who are only somewhat overweight.

The best way to judge whether your weight is endangering your own health is by calculating your body mass index (BMI). This is a scientific formula that uses your height and weight to create an index of just how healthy your weight is; researchers use BMI measurements when studying the prevalence of disease in overweight and obese populations. To calculate your BMI, simply look at the point where your height and weight meet on the chart on the following page. A BMI below 25 means you're at low risk for disease; 25 to 29 puts you at moderately increased risk, and if your BMI is 30 or above, you're at the highest risk.

Your BMI may not sound like good news, but as you lose weight you'll find that the chart can give you incentive to continue: as you progress with the makeover, check back with this chart and you'll be able to watch, week by week, as your health steadily improves.

Determining your BMI will also reveal just how high your risk is for developing certain health conditions. The following findings are based on a 1998 report on the health hazards of being overweight, issued by the National Heart, Lung and Blood Institute in the United States. This is crucial information, demonstrating that losing weight is important not just to help you look better, but to help you avoid serious health risks. Consider this all as good news: losing excess pounds can actually help you avoid many of the greatest risks to your health.

Body Mass Index Table (BMI)

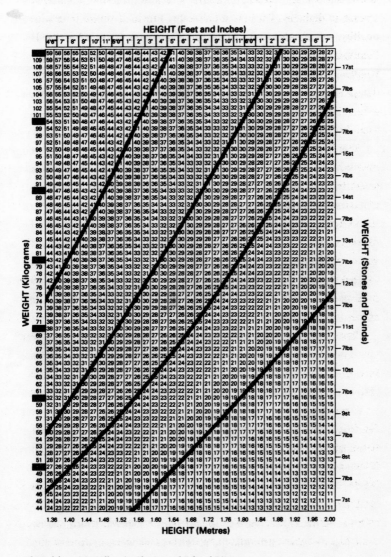

Adapted from J.S. Gallow in *Obesity and Related Diseases*

Hypertension Your risk of high blood pressure increases with every excess pound you carry. If you have a BMI of 30 or greater, you have a 38 per cent risk of developing high blood pressure if you're a man and 32 per cent if you're a woman; men and women whose BMI is under 30, in contrast, have only an 18 per cent and 17 per cent chance, respectively.

High cholesterol Higher body weight is directly associated with high cholesterol levels. Your levels of HDL ('good' cholesterol) drop as you gain weight, while your LDL ('bad' cholesterol) and triglycerides (which should never rise above moderate levels) rise. If you carry more fat around your abdomen (compared to your hips), you may also be at higher risk for having high cholesterol.

Diabetes Recent studies have found that gaining just 11 pounds or more after age eighteen increases your risk of developing Type 2 diabetes. Specifically, your risk of diabetes increases by about 25 percent for every 1 unit increase in your BMI above 22.

Heart disease Your risk of suffering a heart attack or developing heart disease increases even with modest increases in your weight. Researchers found that moderately overweight women (with BMIs of 25 to 28) had twice the risk of developing heart disease and that obese women (with BMIs of 29 or greater) had three times the risk compared to women who weren't overweight.

Stroke Recent studies have shown that your risk of suffering a stroke increases with your weight. If your BMI is greater than 27, you have a 75 per cent higher risk of suffering a stroke; if it's greater than 32, you have a 137 per cent higher risk compared to slender women, according to one study.

Arthritis People who carry around excess weight, not surprisingly, are far more likely to develop knee pain caused by arthritis. One recent study tracked sets of middle-aged female twins in which one twin had developed arthritis; the arthritic twins were on average about 3–5kg (7–11lb) heavier than their sisters. The researchers estimated that for every 1–1.5kg (2–3lb) increase in weight (one BMI unit), an overweight woman's risk of developing arthritis increases by 9 to 13 per cent. By the same token, a decrease in weight of two BMI units or more decreases the odds of developing arthritis in the knee by 50 per cent.

Cancer Being overweight has been linked directly with various forms of cancer. For example, if you are a woman with a BMI of 29 or more, you have twice the risk of developing colon cancer as a woman with a BMI of less than 21. If you tend to have more fat around your abdomen than around your hips, you have a higher risk of developing colon polyps, which can be precursors to cancer. Likewise, studies have shown that being obese increases your risk of dying from postmenopausal breast cancer; gaining just 9kg (20lb) from age eighteen to midlife doubles your risk of breast cancer. And women with a BMI of 30 or more have three times more risk of developing endometrial cancer (cancer of the uterine lining) than a woman who is not overweight.

Restoring Balance to Your Body and Life

As you're probably beginning to realize, you can put yourself in the driving seat when it comes to improving your health. When you make the decision to replace your old eating habits with a new, healthy lifestyle, what you're doing is taking charge of your future. You're taking the necessary steps to restore the balance that's missing from your body and life.

Imagine for a moment that you're living a different life. You eat moderate amounts of food throughout the day, so you never get too hungry and never feel too stuffed. You give your body a wide variety of nutrients in the perfect amounts to keep you healthy, fit and energized. You exercise your heart and muscles and work to improve your flexibility. You've learned to take time out to relax; you feel better about yourself, and your new-found confidence shows through every day in your dealings with others. You take pleasure in your fit new body and revel in the fact that you're living a healthier life.

This is no fantasy. This can be your future, if you're ready to give yourself the Slim•Fast Makeover. It will show you how to eat nutritiously and get the maximum pleasure from the food you eat – without overindulging. You'll learn how to fit exercise into your schedule (no matter how busy you are) and how to choose activities you enjoy, so you'll always *want* to do them. And you'll learn how to relax and take a step back from life's little irritations, helping you focus on achieving your goals. If you nurture your body *and* your mind, you'll reap the ultimate reward: the life you've always wanted.

Taking Charge of Your Health – With Slim•Fast

In the hectic world you live in, you may not have much time to eat properly. If you're running late in the morning, you may skip breakfast. Feeling famished in the late morning, you might be tempted to grab a bar of chocolate or a bag of crisps while on the run. Lunch might consist of one long snack session from afternoon until evening. Dinner might be the only time you sit down and have a real meal – probably thrown together with whatever ingredients you happen to have on hand. Whatever your eating habits, chances are you don't think too hard about what you put into your mouth. You certainly don't have a computer in your head calculating all the calories, fat, vitamins, minerals and nutrients in every morsel you eat.

Unless you're carefully plotting out every meal to ensure that you're getting a properly balanced variety of foods and an ample supply of fruits and vegetables, you're probably lacking many of the essential nutrients your body needs. What's more, when you try to control the foods you eat, you're probably underestimating the number of calories you're really eating in any meal or snack. That's why the Slim•Fast Plan was created – to help people get the nutrition a body needs, while controlling the number of calories they consume.

At the core of the plan are the Slim•Fast shakes, snack bars and meal replacement bars – a line of food products that, when consumed on a regular basis, help you get the fuel your body needs. Unlike some other diet products, Slim•Fast contains no appetite suppressants, 'fat burners', or other additives that claim to speed weight loss. The Slim•Fast meal replacements and snacks are pure food – protein, dietary fibre, a healthy measure of carbohydrates and fat, and up to twenty-four essential vitamins and minerals – more than most people get with three full meals a day, with far fewer calories. Just two shakes (or four meal replacement bars) per day provide you with most of the vitamins and minerals you need to stay healthy.

Unlike liquid diets, the Slim•Fast Plan combines these products with a sensible meal and three snacks, so you won't miss out on the hundreds of nutrients that are found only in fruits, vegetables, fish and whole grains. Combining the shakes with the several daily servings of fruits and vegetables on the plan will enable you to get the **recommended 18 to 30 grams of fibre** each day. Eating this much fibre lowers your risk of colon cancer and heart disease, and has the added advantage of keeping you feeling full between meals, so you won't be as tempted to sneak those snacks in between.

Of course, losing excess weight goes hand in hand with improving your health. And the Slim•Fast Makeover is designed to help you do both. To lose weight on the eating plan, you simply combine two Slim•Fast shakes (or four meal replacement bars) each day with a sensible meal and two or three snacks; then, to maintain your ideal weight once you've reached it, you can switch to one shake a day (or two meal replacement bars) with two sensible meals and snacks. As you'll see in the chapters to come, each meal should contain a healthy serving of protein, a salad, several servings of vegetables, a light serving of starch, and some fruit for dessert. The result is a plan you can live with – and live healthier than ever.

The Slim•Fast Plan has been rigorously tested in clinical trials throughout the world. In one study involving a hundred participants, researchers at an obesity clinic found that Slim•Fast worked better at taking off weight than their subjects' usual diet of traditional foods. At the University of Ulm in Germany, volunteers who used two Slim•Fast meal replacements with a sensible meal and snacks every day for twelve weeks lost an average of over 6kg (15lb). Those who simply tried to cut their intake to between 1,200 and 1,500 calories a day of regular food (by counting calories themselves) lost only 1.5kg (3lb).

In a larger study conducted by David Heber, M.D., Ph.D., director of the UCLA Center for Human Nutrition in the United States, 300 participants followed the Slim•Fast Plan for twelve weeks to lose weight and then continued to use Slim•Fast for two years to maintain their weight loss. Of those who started, 91 per cent completed the first twelve weeks for weight loss; among them, men lost an average of 8.5kg (19lb), women an average of 6kg (14lb). Three-quarters of the subjects continued the weight-maintenance part of the study. After two years, 51 per cent of those participants stayed with the programme: the men maintained an average weight loss of 6.3kg (14lb), the women 6.1kg (13.6lb).

So just following the Slim•Fast eating guidelines alone is a proven way to help you lose weight and maintain the loss for life. And yet there's so much more to the Slim•Fast Makeover than just eating right. By following the exercise and relaxation components of the plan as outlined in these pages, you'll find ways to boost your health and fitness even further – giving yourself every advantage in the great fitness challenge.

Making the Exercise Connection

Until the latter half of the twentieth century, few people had to worry about getting enough exercise. They moved all day long without even thinking about it, walking to and from work, doing heavy manual jobs or laborious housework. However, in the car-driven, remote-control and keyboard world in which we now live, we actually have to *work* to lead an active lifestyle. We schedule in exercise by joining gyms or buying the latest workout videos. Still, most of us quit our exercise programmes within six months of starting them.

Why is it so hard to make exercise part of our lives? The same reason it's so difficult to exercise successfully: we treat both diet and exercise as a means to an end. If we work out hard enough, we tell ourselves, we'll have the body we want. Trouble is, most of us can't possibly work out hard enough to attain the super-sleek figures we see on TV. (Most of those models are born with those bodies – or their managers force them to work out two or three hours a day to achieve them!) When we don't see the results we want right away, most of us get frustrated and quit. And let's face it: exercise can seem like a chore – something to get out of the way before we can get on with what we really want to do. It's the easiest thing in the world to put off, the hardest regime to stick with.

The exercise plan on the Slim•Fast Makeover challenges you to rethink your attitudes to exercise. It offers a wide variety of exercise options, as well as strategies to help you squeeze in activity throughout your day. The one requirement is that you choose an activity that you actually *enjoy*, and stick to it. Maybe you get a buzz from cycling, or hiking, or swimming. If you're having fun and feel energized after your workouts, you won't even think about quitting. After all, how many of us have trouble getting ourselves roused to hit the beach in the summer, or head off on a long walk while we're on holiday? If you can find a few fun things you enjoy doing on a regular basis, get in the habit of doing them regularly and actively, and soon you'll find that exercise has become a part of your life you just can't live without.

The exercise component of the Slim•Fast Makeover calls for you to shift your body into active mode for one hour every day. Now, a full hour may sound like a lot, but if you break it down into smaller chunks – a fifteen-minute walk here, half an hour of biking after work – you should find it more than manageable. You'll also be breaking your workouts down into three different fitness areas: flexibility (stretches), strength (resistance training) and cardiovascular (steady movement like running, walking and swimming). This combination will help you achieve a healthy, fit body. You'll shed fat and put on muscle, which will turn your body into a calorie-burning machine. You'll soon see that the exercise plan works hand in hand with the Slim•Fast eating plan to help maximize your weight-loss efforts. You'll also experience these other amazing health benefits:

You'll be able to shed fat more easily Steady exercise burns off excess calories, which can mobilize your fat cells to release fat, while at the same time a serious workout will elevate your metabolism for several hours after a workout, helping suppress your appetite temporarily. Strength training builds up muscle cells, which use more energy than fat cells, retraining your body to burn calories more quickly and efficiently – that is, triggering your body's natural weight-loss mechanism.

You'll be happier with your body Sedentary people who begin to regularly participate in exercise experience an improved body image and improved self-esteem. This is because the tangible results of regular workout – whether it's increased muscle definition or an improvement in performance – help people recognize their progress.

You'll have an easier time keeping the weight off It is widely recognized that those who keep up their regular exercise routine are far more likely to maintain their weight loss than those who do not.

You can turn back the clock and reverse some signs of ageing Stretching can help counteract the loss of flexibility that occurs as the ageing process begins to shorten your muscle fibres and tendons. As your body begins to be able to move more freely, you'll be helping yourself avoid lower-back and knee injuries, which occur more commonly as you get older. Strength training can also help you turn back the clock. One study found that elderly people who worked out with weights were able to increase their muscle mass at the same rate as twenty-five-year-olds on the same weight-training regime.

Taking a Daily Relaxation Break

How many times have you dug into the biscuit tin to soothe you when you're stressed? How many times has a bar of chocolate served as a little 'pick-me-up' when you're feeling down? All too often, you may turn to food when you're really not that hungry. Maybe you've had a particularly tense day, or you just can't lift yourself out of a slump. Maybe you're just feeling bored and need a dose of instant pleasure.

For years, researchers have been studying the link between food and mood. Researcher Judith Wurtman, Ph.D., of the Massachusetts Institute of Technology in the United States found that cookies and other starchy carbohydrates boost the feel-good brain chemical serotonin; she believes this may explain why women who suffer from premenstrual mood swings crave these snack foods. Other research indicates that chocolate can have mood-enhancing effects because it contains chemicals called cannabinoids – the same class of chemicals that produces a marijuana high. Regardless of whether your food cravings are biochemical or based on habits you learned as a child (like getting a biscuit to soothe a scraped knee), they could be a stumbling block on your road to weight loss. The truth is, when you feel your spirits are flagging, a burst of nutritional energy – the kind you can get from a Slim•Fast snack bar – is a far better idea.

The Slim•Fast Makeover will teach you how to deal with life's little ups and downs without turning to food. You'll set aside twenty minutes a day to get your body into a state of total relaxation. Think of this as a mini-holiday you can take every single day, a pocket of time to take a break from your hectic world.

This plan works in concert with the eating and exercise plans to help you lose weight by managing stress in healthier ways. Like the exercise plan, the relaxation programme offers a variety of techniques, allowing you to choose the one that works best for you. The aim is to feel refreshed after a long day, and renewed for the day you'll be facing tomorrow. You'll find yourself looking forward to your 'away time' every day – that little slice of time when you can put away your cares and concentrate on your happiness.

This relaxation plan may sound a little New Age-y, but it's well known that relaxation can have a host of health benefits – from lowering your risk of heart disease to curing insomnia. Relaxation also lowers your body's production of stress hormones, which are thought to trigger food cravings by throwing your blood sugar levels out of balance. On the flip side, relaxation boosts your brain's production of the 'happy' chemicals, serotonin and endorphins. In short, taking some time daily to relax can help you get the same mellow, pleasurable feeling you may be accustomed to getting from a big piece of chocolate cake. And wouldn't you feel better knowing that you're relaxing *and* helping remake your body, all at once?

Setting Your Weight-Loss Goal

Before you can embark on a weight-loss programme, you need to decide how much weight you want to lose. This can be pretty tricky, considering that the more weight you lose, the greater the chance that you'll gain it all back. This may seem like a cruel trick of nature, but it's actually common sense: the less you weigh, the fewer calories your body needs to maintain your new weight. In other words, if you go from 82kg (12½ stones) down to 54kg (8½ stones), your body – which needed 2,700 calories per day to maintain your heavier weight – will now need only 1,800. That's a whopping 900 calories a day difference between your old and your new eating habits – the equivalent of a hefty lunch in a restaurant. On the other hand, if you go from 82kg (12½ stones) to 68kg (10½ stones), your body will need only 450 fewer calories each day to maintain your weight – a cutback most people should be able to achieve simply by keeping an eye on their portions.

Remember: losing the weight is only half the battle. Maintaining the loss is what wins the war.

Write down your weight-loss goal: _____

The rate at which you'll lose weight will vary depending on how much you currently weigh. The Slim•Fast eating plan contains 1,400–1,500 calories per day – about 1,000 calories fewer than many people normally eat. The ideal rate of weight loss is 0.5–1kg (1–2lb) per week. If you are losing weight much faster than that, you should try adding an extra snack to your eating plan.

The basic fact of weight gain and loss is this: in order to lose weight, you must take in fewer calories than you burn. There are two ways to reach this goal. You can eat fewer calories, or you can increase the calories you burn through exercise. The Slim•Fast Makeover is designed to combine the two strategies – cutting your calories *and* burning off calories through exercise – with a relaxation plan to help you gain control over those weak moments when overindulgence can sabotage even your best efforts.

Ready to get started? Before we begin, let's take a look at how the Slim•Fast Makeover has changed the lives of countless Slim•Fast users.

2

before and after:
Slim•Fast success stories

Every day, millions of people around the world use Slim•Fast products to help them lose weight, feel energized, and feel better about themselves. Over the years, the makers of Slim•Fast have received thousands of letters from consumers who have tried the plan and found that it has actually slimmed their bodies, improved their health – even changed their lives. Countless people have been motivated to begin exercising after losing weight with Slim•Fast. They've remade their eating habits, finding ways to include more fruits and vegetables into their meals and snacks. Very often they've coupled their weight-loss efforts with an exercise programme that has helped them build muscle and stay fit and trim. Some letter writers have even found that Slim•Fast has given them the confidence to make major life changes – from trying out a new career to renewing their passion for an old hobby.

The key to success lies in making Slim•Fast part of a healthy lifestyle. In every one of these success stories, people managed to overcome the habits that kept them overweight, while incorporating new habits to keep themselves slender. What's interesting is that they all took the time to discover what worked best for them. Most remain on Slim•Fast to maintain their weight loss; others turn back to Slim•Fast to take off the extra kilo that they gain from time to time. All of these committed dieters have resolved to live healthy by exercising, eating nutritious foods and taking other steps to improve their lives. And, as their letters reveal, now that they've remade their bodies, they're really enjoying life!

Another advantage of the Slim•Fast approach to weight loss is just how easy it is to use. Many dieters have found that having ready access to Slim•Fast's delicious shakes and bars – whether on the go or after a long day at work – makes it easier for them to stick to the plan instead of giving in to the temptations of fast or processed foods. One such success story is Ann Fields:

After having two children, I finally decided to take off the pounds. I choose Slim•Fast. It made life easy. I didn't have to worry about measuring, mixing or weighing food. I took Slim•Fast in the morning, in the afternoon and then ate a normal dinner. Once you see progress and how much weight you've lost, your goal becomes much more realistic. It was easy for me, I had more energy than I ever had before, I exercised more.

I knew I was on the right track when I could fit into a dress that I bought for a wedding. It was two sizes too small and I said I was going to fit into it whether it was the last thing I did. I looked great! Slim•Fast became a way of life. I use Slim•Fast now in the morning as a breakfast substitute, then I eat a normal lunch and a normal dinner. I know how to regulate my eating so that I can basically still eat what I want. I don't worry about losing weight. It's wonderful, it's healthy. Slim•Fast is part of my life now.

Sometimes losing weight can bring you closer to your family or friends – especially if they act as your support system by encouraging your weight-loss efforts. You may even want to find someone to team up with. Not only can you then support each other in your weight-loss efforts but it can also help you stay committed to your exercise plan if that someone is depending on you to show up for a workout. Bruce Mack found that going through the Slim•Fast Makeover with his wife made losing weight fun and easy. And they got an added bonus: a stronger, happier marriage.

I was truly on the road to self-destruction. Since our marriage in April 1994, my wife, Leslie, and I had progressively gained weight. We couldn't bear to miss our nightly dessert and sometimes an extra helping of something. As my weight soared to a personal record of 254 pounds, I couldn't face my reflection in the mirror. Ultimately, we agreed that Slim•Fast and teamwork offered the greatest promise. Just nine months later, we're both in the best shape of our adult lives! I lost a total of 65 pounds and my wife lost 35 pounds. We have embraced the Slim•Fast process.

My wife and I work in the same building and spend lunch hours together whenever possible – enjoying a leisurely lunch of Slim•Fast at a nearby park before taking an invigorating walk. Once our weight decreased and our spirits increased, we began a serious exercise plan. We now have a fitness room at home with a treadmill and a variety of weights and truly cannot remember when we felt better.

Most successful Slim•Fast users find that exercise speeds their weight loss and helps keep the pounds off. They also see that a combination of exercise and good eating habits gives them more energy and makes them feel healthier. Here's what Dinah Miller Burnette had to say about exercise:

I had been thin all my life – until five years ago. When my doctor prescribed a medication for an unrelated ailment, she warned me that I might gain weight as a side effect but at that point in my life weight was the last thing I was worried about. Over the next two years I gained about 60 pounds but it was so gradual I really didn't notice. Reality finally hit me when I realized I weighed 245 pounds. I woke up and said, I want my old body back.

At first, I bought the Slim•Fast powder and would make myself a shake using just the powder and milk, but then I learned to make wonderful shakes using added ingredients such as fruit. I drank two shakes a day, one for breakfast and one for dinner, and ate a very low-fat meal in the middle of the day.

For exercise, I could only walk one mile a day. I was so heavy that my chest and legs ached very badly. In two months, I lost about 20 pounds, and I was very excited. The more I moved, the more I lost. I was learning the secret: get up, move, and eat right.

Five months after I started losing weight, I had lost almost 50 pounds and was advised to start light weight lifting to tone and firm my body. A fitness instructor started me on a shaping and toning regime, and I also discovered aerobics.

A year and a half has gone by and I've lost 101 pounds, but I feel better than I used to be at this size because I'm exercising and eating right. I have discovered that it's not enough to be thin – you have to be active at whatever size you are.

For some people, the Slim•Fast Makeover has even opened the door to a new career, giving them the confidence and motivation they needed to launch themselves into a new stage of life. Linda Adams is one of those.

After my husband passed away two years ago it was necessary that I go back to work. They weren't exactly beating down the door to hire a sixty-year-old woman back into the hotel business. For professional reasons and to regain my self-esteem, I embarked on a self-improvement programme. When I'm at home, I prepare my Slim•Fast and a banana each morning for breakfast. On the road I freeze a can of Slim•Fast, and by the time it thaws out I'm ready for my lunch drink.

In a year and a half, I've gone from 196 to 139 pounds, returned to work as director of sales and marketing in a hotel, and have again assembled a career wardrobe. I love salads and usually get hungry around 2:00 P.M., so I indulge in my favourite salad. I eat what I want, but only half as much as I used to. I also keep an eye on fat content.

I walk and ride my bike nearly every day for two miles. I feel great, and my five grandchildren think I'm thirty-seven. My friends are in absolute awe of the transformation.

Now that you know the basics of the Slim•Fast Makeover and you've seen how it has helped other dieters achieve the body, mind and life they want, it's time to make a decision. Are you ready to give yourself a makeover? Only you can decide when you're ready to make a change, but getting started sooner is almost always easier than putting things off until 'just the right moment'.

Put a little trust in yourself. You won't let yourself down.

3

14 days to a new you!

When NASA's engineers designed the Apollo 11 spacecraft, they had one central challenge: they had to launch the craft with enough speed and power so that it would not only lift off the ground, but break free from the Earth's gravitational pull. Well, if you can think of your body as the rocket, the Slim•Fast 14-Day Plan is the fuel that will blast you off to weight loss and good health. The initial momentum you'll build on the 14-Day Plan will give you the speed you need to help you reach your ultimate goal: a healthy weight and a healthy body. Once you get that momentum going, you'll see how easy it is to change your life forever.

The point of the 14-Day Plan is to show you how great you can feel once you start eating nutritious foods, exercising and managing the stress in your life. Each of these three components works together to maximize your weight-loss efforts, while improving your health at the same time.

How Much Weight Will You Lose?

Although weight loss varies from person to person, you can lose up to 1–2kgs (3–4lb) while you're on the 14-Day Plan. Assuming that you normally eat around 2,500 calories a day, the plan trims off 1,000–1,100 calories, getting you down to a reasonable intake of 1,400–1,500. And here's how it works: since the average dieter loses about half a kilogram (1 pound) of fat for every 3,500 calories burned, reducing your intake by 1,000 calories a day will enable you to shed half a kilogram (1 pound) every three or four days. And on top of that basic weight loss, most people lose about ½–1kg (1–2lb) of water when they first begin a weight-loss plan. This is because the large amounts of bread, pasta and other starchy carbohydrates we typically eat cause the body to retain excess water, and cutting down on the starches should help you lose a measurable amount of water weight.

Losing 2kg (4lb) in just two weeks can give you the motivation you'll need to continue the healthy habits you began on the 14-Day Plan. And if there's anything that's important in losing weight, it's motivation. That's why the 14-Day Plan is so useful. It can help you start replacing your old habits with a new healthy lifestyle – without any major planning on your part. All you have to do is take your new shopping list to the supermarket, slip into some comfortable exercise clothes for a moderate workout, and follow a lifestyle plan that's enjoyable and rewarding. Soon you'll see that losing weight is more than a dream – it's absolutely within your grasp. Just get your body moving, take some relaxation time for yourself, and follow the simple Slim•Fast eating plan.

Sound Science, No Gimmicks

Sure, the 14-Day Plan sounds great. But how does it work?

The answer is simple: Each of the plan's elements is based on sound science. Slim•Fast meal replacements – Slim•Fast shakes and meal replacement bars – replace the high-calorie meals we're all used to eating with a great-tasting, satisfying alternative. When combined with a sensible meal and snacks, they provide the balanced nutrition you need to feel satisfied and energized on fewer calories. And they contain no appetite suppressants, fat-burning chemicals, or drugs of any kind. The exercise must-dos give you a selection of strategies to help boost your body's metabolism, so you'll burn more calories and lose weight faster. And the instant stress relievers will give you a mini-holiday every day from life's little aggravations – the daily distractions that can sabotage your weight-loss efforts by undermining your motivation and sending you back to the kitchen for another tasty helping of high-calorie comfort food.

The proper balance of nutrition, exercise and relaxation you'll get on the 14-Day Plan will help you balance your body's systems. Your digestive system can run more smoothly, since you'll be eating smaller meals more frequently throughout the day; you'll be less likely to experience heartburn and other symptoms of indigestion, and the added fibre in the Slim•Fast Plan will help prevent constipation. You may also experience more energy as your body becomes better at absorbing the balanced level of nutrients in your diet – and as your circulation improves through exercise and relaxation.

In short, your body will finally be working for you instead of against you – retraining itself, through your new lifestyle, to help you live the life you want.

14 Days of Eating Right

The Slim•Fast Plan, with its basic 1,400- to 1,500-calorie daily allowance, is simple and easy to follow. It also gives you the most nutritious foods for the fewest amount of calories. Unlike many other calorie-restricted diets, which require you to guesstimate the number of calories you're consuming, the Slim•Fast Plan takes away the guesswork and enables you to eat the actual number of calories on the plan. (Note: the precise nutritional content of products varies according to the variety of product used.)

At the centre of the plan is the balanced, medically proven combination of vitamins, minerals and other nutrients that goes into every Slim•Fast product. Each day on the plan you'll be drinking two great-tasting Slim•Fast shakes (or eating four meal replacement bars) plus a Slim•Fast snack bar between meals. One shake provides one-third of your daily requirements for most vitamins and minerals. It also provides the right amounts of fibre, protein and carbohydrates, along with a small amount of fat, for a total of 200–220 calories. The meal-replacement system gives you a way to get the nutrients you need, with a limited number of calories, without depriving you of the pleasures of eating. And the proper balance of nutrients in Slim•Fast products will help your body absorb nutrients more efficiently.

But don't worry, there's more to the eating plan than just shakes and bars. The 14-Day Plan includes a sensible dinner every night and provides for snacking throughout the day – a programme based on sensible dietary guidelines established by the U.S. Department of Agriculture. These guidelines call for eating a variety of foods in order to get the forty nutrients (such as vitamins, minerals, protein and fibre) that are essential for good health. And they emphasize that no single food can provide all the nutrients in the amounts you need. They recommend that 30 per cent or less of your total daily calories come from fat, that 20 per cent of your calories come from protein, and that 50 per cent come from carbohydrates (fruits, vegetables, starches etc.).

To help you meet those guidelines every day, each day of the 14-Day Plan includes a series of recipes and snacking suggestions – featuring several servings of vegetables as well as a fibre-rich starch. The recipes also contain ample amounts of lower-fat proteins such as fish, white-meat poultry, lean cuts of meat, and pulses. Oils and other fats are used sparingly, and fresh fruit is featured for dessert.

Combine these dinners with two Slim•Fast meal-replacement shakes (or four meal replacement bars), three fresh fruit snacks and a Slim•Fast snack bar, and your total calorie intake for the day will be around 1,400–1,500 calories. This is a perfect eating plan for losing weight slowly and steadily – on the order of ½–1kg (1–2lb) a week. That's the safest and most effective way to lose weight, according to health experts.

The 14-Day Plan also emphasizes another major nutrient: fibre. Fibre helps combat such health ills as colorectal cancer, gastrointestinal disorders, diabetes and heart disease – and, because it makes you feel full more quickly, fibre can also help you curb overeating. Each Slim•Fast shake contains up to 5 grams of fibre; two shakes plus the fruits, vegetables and grains recommended on the plan will make it easy to meet the recommended daily intake of 18–30 grams. In simple terms, the 14-Day Plan will very likely have you eating better than you have in years. After all, most of us eat fewer than five servings of fruits and vegetables a day and don't come close to ingesting the recommended amount of fibre. When you consider that you're probably not getting enough calcium and other essential vitamins and minerals – or enough phytochemicals, the disease-fighting nutrients found in fruits and vegetables – you'll realize how much you have to gain from trying the plan.

The 14-Day Plan will also teach you cooking tricks to help you save on fat and calories. The recipes all emphasize healthy cooking techniques: foods are grilled, steamed and baked – not fried. Nonstick low-calorie cooking sprays are used to coat pans instead of oil. Dressings for salads are fat-free or reduced-calorie. The protein choices include lean cuts of meat, white-meat chicken and turkey, and fish, to help you get the greatest helpings of nutrients with the least amount of saturated fat. Vegetables are a prominent part of every meal, and fruit plays a starring role at dessert.

Here's a quick rundown of the plan you'll be following. It's been tested by millions of Slim•Fast users, and it works!

To help you lose weight, the plan calls for you to replace two regular meals a day with Slim•Fast shakes or meal replacement bars; to snack lightly throughout the day on fruit, vegetables, or Slim•Fast snack bars; and to finish it all off with a sensible dinner. Here's the basic Weight-Loss Plan:

TO LOSE WEIGHT, JUST REMEMBER:

Shake • Shake • Meal

BREAKFAST: 1 Slim•Fast Shake or 2 Meal Replacement Bars
SNACK: 1 piece of fruit or 115g/4oz raw vegetables
LUNCH: 1 Slim•Fast Shake or 2 Meal Replacement Bars
SNACK: 1 piece of fruit or 115g/4oz raw vegetables
SNACK: 1 Slim•Fast Snack Bar or 1 serving very low fat yogurt
DINNER: 1 large tossed salad; 170g/6oz of protein (meat, chicken, fish, or soya/vegetable protein); 3 servings of cooked or steamed vegetables; 1 serving of starch (½ baked potato, 1 small corn on the cob, or 85g/3oz rice or pasta); 1 piece of fruit for dessert

Important: On the Slim•Fast Plan, it's crucial to drink eight glasses of water each day to keep your body hydrated. You can still drink caffeinated coffee, tea, or diet colas, but don't count them toward your water amount because the caffeine they contain tends to dehydrate the body.

Once you've finished losing the weight you want – whether it's the two kilograms you lost on the 14-Day Plan or another ten you lost by staying on the plan until you reached your goal – it's important to keep up your efforts. The Slim•Fast Plan makes it easy to keep your weight in check with the Weight Maintenance Plan, which calls for two sensible meals and one shake or two meal replacement bars per day.

TO MAINTAIN YOUR IDEAL WEIGHT, REMEMBER:

Meal • Shake • Meal

BREAKFAST: 1 bowl (30g/1oz) high-fibre cereal; 125ml/4fl oz skimmed milk; 115g/4oz very low fat yogurt; 1 piece fruit; or 1 Slim•Fast Shake or 2 Meal Replacement Bars

SNACK: 1 piece of fruit

LUNCH: 55g/2oz cold meat or cheese; 3 servings vegetables (lettuce, grated carrots, tomato slices, etc.); 2 slices wholemeal bread; 225g/8oz very low fat yogurt, ½ melon; or 1 Slim•Fast Shake or 2 Meal Replacement Bars

SNACK: 1 piece of fruit

SNACK: 1 Slim•Fast Snack Bar or 1 serving very low fat yogurt

DINNER: Vegetable soup or side salad; 170g/6oz protein (meat, chicken, fish, or soya/vegetable protein); 3 servings of cooked or steamed vegetables; 1 serving of starch (potato, rice, pasta, etc.); 1 piece of fruit for dessert

Weighing in – Every Day

In recent years, the scale has gotten a bad reputation. Many obesity experts warned that people had become too obsessed with the bottom-line number on the scale instead of focusing on healthy habits that would help them lose weight naturally.

But the fact is, a weight scale remains one of the most useful tools we have in the effort to maintain control of our weight. It's cheap to buy, convenient to use – and it doesn't lie. During the 14-Day Plan you should make it a point to weigh yourself every day – and it's a habit you should continue even after finishing the plan. Weighing yourself every day provides an instant way to monitor your efforts. If you see the scale begin to inch up, you can immediately cut back on calories or step up your physical activity. You'll then be able to set yourself back on track before you find yourself stepping into a larger pair of trousers.

Fit, Fabulous and Fun

Along with the mouth-watering menus that feature in the 14-Day Plan, each day includes what we call an exercise must-do. These exercises are designed to give you a mixture of cardiovascular activity (steady exercise that works your heart muscle and makes you sweat), resistance training (toning exercises to strengthen your muscles), and stretching techniques (exercises that increase flexibility and balance). The exercises change every day, so you won't get bored doing the same thing over and over; there's something to suit everyone's tastes to help you find the exercises you enjoy most – and thus will be most likely to come back to on a permanent basis.

The goal of the exercise portion of the plan is to get your body moving for an hour every day. That might sound like a lot at first but if you break it up into manageable mini-workouts throughout the day, you can accomplish a lot even if you can't steal a full hour away. And it's even easier if you can find ways to walk or cycle instead of driving during the course of your regular day. So supplement the exercise tips on the 14-Day Plan with a little moving of your own. Whether it's bopping around the house to your favourite CD or running around the garden with your kids, you should be having fun and getting active at the same time.

You might ask: do I really need to exercise if I can lose weight on the Slim•Fast Plan alone? For your answer, consider some of the health benefits of exercise:

Increases metabolic rate It's one of the paradoxes of dieting: the less you eat and the less you weigh, the lower your metabolism – the rate at which your body burns calories. Thus, you need to eat less to maintain your loss, and even less to keep losing weight. Exercise helps counteract this problem by speeding up your metabolism – during your workouts and for several hours afterwards.

Counteracts the health ills of obesity Exercise can help alleviate many of the health problems that come with being overweight. It can reduce your risk of heart disease by improving blood pressure and cholesterol levels. It can help stabilize blood sugar and reduce insulin resistance, to lower your risk of diabetes. It gives you energy by improving the circulation of your blood. And by strengthening your muscles, it helps alleviate joint problems that result from carrying too much excess weight.

Helps control appetite Studies with both animals and humans suggest that exercise can help control appetite – at least when you work out moderately. Unfortunately, many of us tend to reward ourselves after a workout with 'just a taste' of the wrong kind of food – and it takes only a few biscuits to add back the calories you just burned. Beware the urge to splurge – that's your mind talking, not your body.

Preserves the body's muscle The fact is, your body tends to lose muscle as well as fat when you lose weight. Exercise can help maximize fat loss while limiting muscle loss; combining exercise with diet does this more effectively than diet alone.

Improves confidence and psychological factors There's no quicker route to a better body image – and greater confidence – than exercise. Just the fact that you're making positive changes can boost your spirits, and as you see your body becoming more toned and fit your self-confidence is sure to follow. Research also suggests that exercise helps at the hormonal level, increasing your 'feel-good' endorphins and reducing stress hormones. Exercise can also be a great stress reliever if you're used to eating when you're tense – and that can only bolster your weight-loss efforts.

Increases your chances of long-term success Studies show that exercise is the most important factor in determining how well dieters maintain weight loss. It's simple: stay with the exercise programme and you'll help those pounds stay off.

Nurture Yourself

The third element of the 14-Day Plan is the instant stress reliever included for each day of the plan. The truth is, the only smart way to remake your body and life is to pay equal attention to remaking your mind – taking the time to care for the inner you. It might surprise you that a weight-loss plan would devote much time to something as natural as relaxation; after all, most of us lead such busy lives that we'd never dream we'd need help to learn to relax. After all, you might think, who needs lessons in relaxation if I already spend an hour or two every night vegging out in front of the TV?

Once you've tried the relaxation techniques on the 14-Day Plan, though, you'll realize the difference between being a couch potato and practising high-quality relaxation. The best relaxation leaves you feeling refreshed because you've taken the time to focus on clearing your head of your daily stresses and releasing the tensions that you've built up over the course of a stressful day. Instead of settling for sneaking half an hour of rest in between tense moments – distracting yourself for half an hour with a magazine, say, before getting up to make dinner – on the 14-Day Plan you'll learn to free yourself from your daily tensions and renew your spirit.

One other important fact to remember is the importance of sleep. Too many of us assume we can get by with as little as five or six hours of sleep a night – going to bed at 12:30 A.M., say, and getting up at 6:30. But the truth is, very few people can function well on that little sleep. Most adults need seven to nine hours a night to achieve optimal rest. Researchers believe that sleep is our body's most important period of rest and recovery, restoring the brain and body after the normal stresses of daily activity. Getting too little sleep can impair your ability to concentrate, cause memory problems and make you feel drowsy and moody throughout the day. Some studies even suggest that getting too little sleep can shorten your life span. Getting the right amount of sleep is essential during the 14-Day Plan. Even if you're following the plan to the letter, you won't get the energy boost you should, or feel as great as you can, if you aren't getting enough sleep.

Now you're ready to begin the 14-Day Plan. It's time to make some sensible changes to your way of living, to improve your health and create a happier life for yourself. It's time to give yourself a makeover – inside and out, body, mind, and life.

So what are you waiting for?

4

the 14-day plan

day 1

Now it's time to put all your good intentions into practice. Use the hopes you have for the future as your motivation – you'll be taking hold of your destiny and making a change that will enable you to look better, feel better and be healthier.

Daily Menu

NOTE: The meals on each day of the plans are interchangeable. If you like some foods better than others, feel free to mix and match: have the dinner from Day 5 again on Day 9, or have one of the dinners for lunch and enjoy a shake when you get home. Just make sure that two of your meals are Slim•Fast shakes or Meal Replacement Bars, and the third is one of the sensible meals from the plan.

BREAKFAST
1 Slim•Fast French Vanilla Powder Shake
    (or your favourite Slim•Fast shake)
Glass of water

MORNING SNACK

225g/8oz virtually fat-free yogurt, artificially sweetened

Glass of water

LUNCH

1 Slim•Fast Ready to Drink Shake

Glass of water

AFTERNOON SNACK

1 Slim•Fast Snack Bar

Glass of water

DINNER
Salad

    55g/2oz mixed lettuce

    55g/2oz mushrooms, sliced

    ½ cucumber, peeled and sliced

    2 tablespoons fat-free dressing

170g/6oz turkey breast meat, grilled and sliced

2 tablespoons cranberry sauce

55g/2oz steamed peas

55g/2oz steamed carrots

55g/2oz steamed broccoli

½ medium baked sweet potato

1 kiwi fruit, sliced

Glass of water

EVENING SNACK

1 pear

Glass of water

day 1 nutritional information

day total	calories	protein	carbs	fat	fibre	sodium	cholesterol	calcium
	1,448	95 g	221 g	24 g (14%)	35 g	1,352 mg	147 mg	1,363 mg

Exercise Must-Do Today, concentrate on getting small bursts of exercise – climb stairs, skip, pedal, or run on an exercise machine for five minutes twice a day. Choose activities that you can do at a moment's notice, and push hard enough to feel worn out when you're finished. Add two ten-minute brisk outdoor walks in the morning and evening, along with a fifteen-minute walk at lunch and you've got a forty-five-minute workout – a great start.

Instant Stress Reliever At the end of the day, write down any of the little tensions that got to you during the day. Next to them, make two columns. In the first column, rate (from 1 to 10) how strongly you reacted to each of them while they were happening; in the second column, rate how important they seem to you now, in retrospect. The very act of putting your stress into perspective should help to relax you.

Daily Weigh-in _____

day 2

While you're carefully following this 14-Day Plan, don't forget to take some time to be spontaneous. Plan a family outing with no destination in mind. Just hop in the car and see where you end up. Let someone else make the plans for the evening and surprise you. By breaking up your old routine you'll be giving yourself a chance to see life from a new perspective.

Daily Menu

BREAKFAST
2 Slim•Fast Meal Replacement Bars (or 1 Slim•Fast shake)
125ml/4fl oz fresh orange juice
Glass of water

MORNING SNACK
1 apple
Glass of water

LUNCH
1 Slim•Fast Ready to Drink Shake
Glass of water

AFTERNOON SNACK
Celery and Carrot Sticks
    1 celery stick, cut into strips
    1 large carrot, cut into strips
Glass of water

DINNER

Spinach Salad

    55g/2oz young spinach, torn into bite-size pieces

    ½ medium red onion, chopped

    55g/2oz very fresh button mushrooms, sliced

    2 tablespoons fat-free dressing

Savoury Grilled Cod (page 38)

85g/3oz steamed white rice

70g/2½oz steamed courgettes

70g/2½oz steamed summer squash

6 steamed asparagus spears

85g/3oz pineapple chunks (in juice) with 2 wholemeal crackers

Glass of water

EVENING SNACK

1 Slim•Fast Snack Bar

Glass of water

day 2 nutritional information

day total	calories	protein	carbs	fat	fibre	sodium	cholesterol	calcium
	1,431	73 g	235 g	25 g (16%)	27 g	1,732 mg	116 mg	1,124 mg

Savoury Grilled Cod

SERVES 4   total preparation time: **12 minutes**

115g/4oz low-calorie mayonnaise
¼ onion, grated or very finely diced
2 tablespoons lemon juice
780g/1¾ lb cod fillet (substitute haddock or other white fish)
1 large tomato, thinly sliced

1. Preheat grill.
2. In a small mixing bowl, combine mayonnaise with grated onion and lemon juice; mix well.
3. Rinse fish and pat dry. Place on a baking tray or grill pan. Spoon mayonnaise sauce over fish to cover, then top with sliced tomato. Grill 6–7 minutes or until fish flakes easily with a fork or becomes translucent.

nutritional information per serving

	calories	protein	carbs	fat	fibre	sodium	cholesterol	calcium
	263	39 g	8 g	7 g (25%)	1 g	286 mg	101 mg	29 mg

Exercise Must-Do If you see an opportunity to get yourself moving, take advantage of it. Park in a space at the far side of the car park and walk; forgo the cleaning lady and clean your house yourself; instead of having a barbecue in the back garden, walk to a picnic spot.

Instant Stress Reliever Sit comfortably and close your eyes. Breathe slowly, becoming aware of the breath passing in and out of your body. Every time you exhale, say the word 'Relax' to yourself. As you say it, let the word take effect on the various parts of your body: untense your forehead, loosen your shoulders, relax your arms and legs. Round your back from the waist and reach toward your toes. Come back up and open your eyes.

Daily Weigh-in _____

day 3

Take ten minutes in the morning to write down one goal that you're setting for yourself today. This should be a character-building goal – the kind of wish that's usually preceded by words such as 'I wish I could be more ...' Today, give yourself permission to act this way – whether it means taking a little more time with your children or saying 'no' to something you don't want to do. Give yourself a day to try on your new self – you can always slip back into your old self tomorrow.

Daily Menu

BREAKFAST
1 Slim•Fast Chocolate Royale Powder Shake
    (or your favourite Slim•Fast shake)
Glass of water

MORNING SNACK
1 orange
Glass of water

LUNCH
2 Slim•Fast Meal Replacement Bars
15 grapes
Glass of water

AFTERNOON SNACK
1 Slim•Fast Snack Bar
Glass of water

DINNER

250ml/8fl oz canned low-fat lentil soup

Wholewheat Pasta with Spinach Pesto (page 42)

Baked Golden Acorn Squash (page 43)

55g/2oz steamed green beans

⅛ honeydew melon

Glass of water

EVENING SNACK

1 medium banana

Glass of water

day 3 nutritional information

day total	calories	protein	carbs	fat	fibre	sodium	cholesterol	calcium
	1,478	61 g	269 g	26 g (16%)	46 g	1,072 mg	31 mg	1,480 mg

Wholewheat Pasta with Spinach Pesto

SERVES 4   total preparation time: **15 minutes**

115g/4oz wholewheat pasta
225g/8oz fresh spinach, stems removed, and shredded
2 cloves garlic, crushed
30g/1oz pine nuts
40g/1½oz grated Parmesan cheese
225g/8oz very low fat natural yogurt
1 tablespoon olive oil

1. Bring a large saucepan of water to the boil, add pasta and cook according to package directions until al dente. Drain, cover and keep warm.
2. Meanwhile, prepare the pesto. In a liquidizer or food processor, combine spinach, garlic, pine nuts, Parmesan cheese, yogurt and olive oil. Blend until puréed.
3. Place cooked pasta in a large shallow serving bowl, top with pesto and mix thoroughly.

nutritional information per serving

	calories	protein	carbs	fat	fibre	sodium	cholesterol	calcium
	364	19 g	50 g	12 g (30%)	8 g	288 mg	11 mg	295 mg

Baked Golden Acorn Squash

SERVES 4   total preparation time: **65 minutes**

Vegetable cooking spray

2 medium acorn squash, halved and seeded

2 tablespoons maple syrup

½ teaspoon ground cinnamon

½ teaspoon granulated artificial sweetener

¼ teaspoon ground black pepper

1. Preheat oven to 180°C/350°F/Gas mark 4.
2. Spray a medium baking tray with vegetable cooking spray. Lay squash halves, cut side down, in the baking tray. Bake, uncovered, until tender when pierced with a fork, 45 minutes.
3. Turn squash halves cut side up. Drizzle maple syrup over squash and sprinkle with cinnamon, sweetener and black pepper. Continue baking until edges are browned, 15 minutes.

nutritional information per serving

calories	protein	carbs	fat	fibre	sodium	cholesterol	calcium
113	2 g	30 g	0.2 g (2%)	3 g	7 mg	0 mg	82 mg

Exercise Must-Do While you're watching TV, tone and strengthen your abdominal muscles and chest by doing some crunches and modified pushups.

To do a crunch, lie on your back with your knees bent and your arms crossed over your chest. While keeping your eyes on your knees, inhale and raise your shoulders and back about five centimetres off the floor. Exhale and lower back to the floor. Do as many as you can.

For a modified pushup, position yourself on your hands and knees, feet up and crossed at the ankles. Place your hands a bit wider apart than your shoulders; keep your arms straight, but don't lock the elbows. Your neck, back and waist should be in a straight line. Pull in your abdominal muscles and slowly lower yourself down until your arms are bent 90 degrees, exhaling as you go. Inhale while pushing yourself up. Do a set of ten, or as many as you can.

Instant Stress Reliever Try giving yourself an aromatherapy oil treatment. This deep conditioning treatment will soften your hair and your mood. Wet your hair and towel it dry until it's lightly damp. In the palm of your hand blend one to three teaspoons of olive oil (more for longer hair, less for shorter) with a few drops of scented lavender or jasmine oil. Massage the mixture into your scalp, working in small circles from your forehead to the base of your neck. Cover your hair with a plastic bag and wrap a towel around that. Relax for twenty minutes. Put your feet up, listen to your favourite CD and drink a cup of herbal tea. Shampoo hair thoroughly and rinse clean.

Daily Weigh-in _____

day 4

Don't hide behind nondescript clothes or hair. Even if you're working on improving your appearance, you should take pride in the way you look right now. Buy yourself a new shirt in the latest colour, or trousers cut in a trendy style (even if you may need a smaller size in a few months). Update your hairstyle. Taking care of yourself sends the world a message: I like myself, and others ought to like me, too.

Daily Menu

BREAKFAST

1 Slim•Fast Strawberry Supreme Powder Shake
    (or your favourite Slim•Fast shake)
Glass of water

MORNING SNACK

1 Slim•Fast Snack Bar
Glass of water

LUNCH
Large Tossed Salad

    30g/1oz cos lettuce, chopped
    30g/1oz iceberg lettuce, chopped
    55g/2oz very fresh button mushrooms, sliced
    1 tomato, quartered
    2 tablespoons fat-free dressing
Fancy Turkey Salad (page 47)
One 15cm/6-inch (40g/1½ oz) pitta bread
15 seedless grapes
Glass of water

AFTERNOON SNACK

225g/8oz virtually fat-free yogurt, artificially sweetened

Glass of water

DINNER

1 Slim•Fast Ready to Drink Shake

10 baby carrots

2 plums

Glass of water

EVENING SNACK

180ml/6fl oz cranberry juice mixed with sparkling mineral water and a
squeeze of fresh lime

Glass of water

day 4 nutritional information

day total	calories	protein	carbs	fat	fibre	sodium	cholesterol	calcium
	1,436	99 g	227 g	18 g (11%)	25 g	1,434 mg	167 mg	1,575 mg

Fancy Turkey Salad

SERVES 4   **total preparation time: 40 minutes**

Vegetable cooking spray
780g/1¾ lb chopped turkey breast meat
2 tablespoons very low fat natural yogurt
2 teaspoons lemon juice
1 tablespoon low-fat mayonnaise
¼ teaspoon onion powder
Dash ground white pepper
2 celery sticks, diced
30g/1oz walnuts, chopped
1 medium apple, cored and diced
1 head red-leaf lettuce, torn into bite-size pieces

1. Spray a large nonstick frying pan with vegetable cooking spray and heat over medium-high heat. Add turkey and sauté, turning frequently, until cooked through, 6–8 minutes.
2. Place cooked turkey on a plate, cover and refrigerate to cool, 10–15 minutes.
3. Meanwhile, in a small mixing bowl, combine yogurt, lemon juice, mayonnaise, onion powder and white pepper. Mix with spoon or whisk until blended.
4. When cool, place turkey meat in a large mixing bowl. Add celery, walnuts and apple, fold in the dressing and gently mix well. Cover and chill in refrigerator 10–15 minutes.
5. Place lettuce leaves on 4 plates and top with dressed turkey salad.

nutritional information per serving

	calories	protein	carbs	fat		fibre	sodium	cholesterol	calcium
	320	54 g	10 g	7 g (18%)		2 g	140 mg	142 mg	62 mg

Exercise Must-Do Take a twenty-minute 'power walk', which burns more calories than regular walking and helps improve your fitness. Walk in short quick strides at a pace that's just below a jog. Pump your arms to work your upper body and increase your calorie burn even more.

Instant Stress Reliever Try 'Bellow's Breath', a yoga breathing exercise. Take a deep breath, inhaling slowly until your lungs feel full. Now exhale for a count of twenty, slowly emptying all the air out of your lungs. Take one final deep breath and then breathe comfortably, focusing on your breathing.

Daily Weigh-in _____

day 5

It may seem surprising but many women overestimate their body size. And the more inaccurate women are about their body size, the worse they feel about themselves. Here's a simple technique that might help you see your body the way it really is. Unravel a ball of string, and make a loop that you think reflects the circumference of your waist. Set that aside. Take another piece of string and do the same for your hips. Now take two more pieces of string and measure the real circumference of your waist and hips. Compare the length of the real measurements with the loops you estimated for your waist and hips. See the difference?

Daily Menu

BREAKFAST

1 Slim•Fast Banana Deluxe Powder Shake
   (or your favourite Slim•Fast shake)
Glass of water

MORNING SNACK

1 tangerine
Glass of water

LUNCH

1 Slim•Fast Ready to Drink Shake
Glass of water

AFTERNOON SNACK

1 Slim•Fast Snack Bar
Glass of water

DINNER

125ml/4fl oz tomato juice

'Good-for-You' Fried Chicken (page 51)

Rice and Beans

    85g/3oz steamed brown rice

    45g/1½ oz canned black beans

    55g/2oz steamed carrots

    115g/4oz steamed spinach

1 nectarine (sliced) with 2 tablespoons low-fat whipped topping

Glass of water

EVENING SNACK

85g/3oz plain air-popped popcorn

Glass of water

day 5 nutritional information

day total	calories	protein	carbs	fat	fibre	sodium	cholesterol	calcium
	1,425	91 g	204 g	29 g (18%)	31 g	1,230 mg	162 mg	1,233 mg

'Good-for-You' Fried Chicken

SERVES 4   **total preparation time: 15 minutes**

780g/1¾ lb boneless, skinless chicken breasts
½ teaspoon paprika
¼ teaspoon salt
½ teaspoon ground black pepper
20g/¾ oz wheat germ
2 teaspoons olive oil

1. Rinse chicken and pat dry. With a meat tenderizer, lightly pound until each breast is 1–1.5cm/⅓–½ inch thick.
2. On a plate, thoroughly mix paprika, salt, pepper and wheat germ. Dip each piece of chicken in the spice mixture to coat evenly, then set aside.
3. Heat the oil in a large nonstick pan over medium-high heat. Add the chicken breasts and sauté 2–3 minutes on each side, until lightly brown and juices run clear when pricked with a fork. Remove from pan and serve immediately.

nutritional information per serving

calories	protein	carbs	fat	fibre	sodium	cholesterol	calcium
383	53 g	4 g	16 g (38%)	1 g	267 mg	143 mg	29 mg

Exercise Must-Do Today, work on increasing your flexibility. Whether you're off for a short hike or a long jog, do this stretch beforehand to loosen up your hamstrings and help prevent injury. Stand and place a chair in front of you. Put one heel on the chair, with the leg extended; lean forward from the hips until you feel gentle resistance. Hold for 30 seconds. Repeat on the other leg.

Instant Stress Reliever One good way to release all the stress and tension stored in your muscles is by practising progressive muscle relaxation. Lie back comfortably and close your eyes. Working your way from your toes to your head, tense each muscle group for two seconds and then release. Curl your toes, hold for two seconds, release. Flex your feet, hold for two seconds, release. Tighten your shins, tense your thighs, scrunch your fingers into a fist, tense your arms, shrug your shoulders, curl your back, purse your lips and tighten your forehead. After you've tensed and released each muscle group, tense them all together and release. Your body should be completely relaxed.

Daily Weigh-in _____

day 6

Today, try silencing any critical voices that might be rattling around in your head. If you call yourself 'thunder thighs' when you're working out, stop. You wouldn't put up with a stranger calling you names, would you? Concentrate on your strengths instead of your perceived shortcomings – it'll help you stay focused on your goal.

Daily Menu

BREAKFAST
1 Slim•Fast Shake, choose your favourite
Glass of water

MORNING SNACK
1 Slim•Fast Snack Bar
Glass of water

LUNCH
2 Slim•Fast Meal Replacement Bars
Celery and Carrot Sticks
    1 celery stick, cut into strips
    1 large carrot, cut into strips
Glass of water

AFTERNOON SNACK
6 virtually fat-free wholemeal crispbreads
Glass of water

DINNER

Salad

   55g/2oz green-leaf lettuce, chopped

   1 tomato, quartered

   55g/2oz green pepper, cored and diced

   2 tablespoons balsamic vinegar

170g/6oz grilled tuna fillet with lemon and dill

15cm/6-inch piece corn on the cob

115g/4oz baked butternut squash

55g/2oz steamed green beans

¼ cantaloupe melon

Glass of water

EVENING SNACK

225g/8oz canned peaches in juice

Glass of water

day 6 nutritional information

day total	calories	protein	carbs	fat		fibre	sodium	cholesterol	calcium
	1,431	88 g	228 g	24 g (15%)		38 g	809 mg	103 mg	1,209 mg

Exercise Must-Do Do a set of bottom-lifters – a quick toning move – at your desk at work. First, with feet together, stand behind a chair and hold on to the back. Lunge back with your right leg, placing the ball of your right foot on the floor. Then, lower the right knee until the left thigh is almost parallel to the floor. Keep the left knee in line above the ankle – don't lean forward. Then return to the starting position. Do 15 repetitions, then repeat on the other leg.

Instant Stress Reliever Here's another easy yoga pose – the cross-legged forward bend. On the floor, sit tall with legs crossed between ankles and shins. Press your fingers into the floor behind you for support. Lengthen your waist and lift your chest. Hold for a minute. Take long, deep breaths, expanding your belly on each inhale, pulling your navel in on each exhale. On an exhale, slowly release torso forward, bending from hips. Rest arms and head on the floor or a pillow. Relax your shoulders and neck, holding for one minute.

Daily Weigh-in _____

day 7

As you continue with the 14-Day Plan, you're doing everything possible to improve your health by eating right, exercising and managing stress. While you're making the most out of your life, spend some time thinking about how you deal with day-to-day problems. Do you have trouble coping when things don't go as expected? Consider finding other ways to cope with trials when they occur.

Daily Menu

BREAKFAST

1 Slim•Fast Strawberry Supreme Powder Shake
    (or your favourite Slim•Fast shake)
Glass of water

MORNING SNACK

1 pear
Glass of water

LUNCH

1 Slim•Fast Ready to Drink Shake
115g/4oz strawberries
Glass of water

AFTERNOON SNACK

½ bagel (85g/3oz) with 1 teaspoon low-fat soft cheese spread
Glass of water

DINNER

Tossed Salad

    55g/1oz cos lettuce, chopped

    55g/1oz iceberg lettuce, chopped

    6 cherry tomatoes

    55g/2oz very fresh button mushrooms, sliced

170g/6oz lean grilled sirloin steak

½ baked potato

115g/4oz steamed broccoli and cauliflower

55g/2oz steamed peas

85g/3oz fruit sorbet with 115g/4oz strawberries

Glass of water

EVENING SNACK

1 Slim•Fast Snack Bar

Glass of water

day 7 nutritional information

day total	calories	protein	carbs	fat	fibre	sodium	cholesterol	calcium
	1,432	97 g	216 g	24 g (15%)	33 g	1,133 mg	172 mg	1,271 mg

Exercise Must-Do Get a real workout without breaking up your daily routine. Instead of strolling to pick up your children from a friend's house, get a real move on. Take the dog for an extra walk instead of playing fetch. Cycle to work instead of driving.

Instant Stress Reliever Give yourself a soothing salt scrub. Combine 450g/1lb of sea salt with 125ml/4fl oz of shower gel in a small bowl until blended. (Don't use table salt; the grains are too small and will melt.) In the shower or bath, splash yourself with warm water and work the salt mixture into your skin using small circular motions. Pay special attention to rough areas like knees, elbows and the soles of your feet. After covering your body, rinse and lightly towel dry, then apply a lavish coat of moisturising body lotion.

Daily Weigh-in _____

day 8

'Happy people are often in a zone called "flow," absorbed in a task that challenges them without overwhelming them,' observed David Myers, Ph.D., author of *The Pursuit of Happiness*. Today, take at least thirty minutes to challenge your mind by doing something different from your usual routine. Play Scrabble, do a tricky crossword puzzle, practise on an instrument you haven't touched in years, or start a home-improvement project you've been putting off.

Daily Menu

BREAKFAST
1 Slim•Fast French Vanilla Powder Shake
    (or your favourite Ultra Slim•Fast shake)
Glass of water

MORNING SNACK
20g packet apple chips (or 20g/¾ oz dried fruit)
250ml/8fl oz diet hot chocolate
Glass of water

LUNCH
2 Slim•Fast Meal Replacement Bars
Celery and Carrot Sticks with Salsa
    1 celery stick, cut into strips
    1 large carrot, cut into strips
    55g/2oz salsa
Glass of water

AFTERNOON SNACK
1 Slim•Fast Snack Bar
Glass of water

DINNER

250ml/8fl oz canned low-fat vegetable soup

Salad Niçoise (recipe below)

30g/1oz wholemeal roll

¼ cantaloupe melon

Glass of water

EVENING SNACK

1 banana

Glass of water

day 8 nutritional information

day total	calories	protein	carbs	fat	fibre	sodium	cholesterol	calcium
	1,500	53 g	243 g	28 g (17%)	30 g	2,521 mg	65 mg	2,222 mg

Salade Niçoise

SERVES 4   **total preparation time: 25 minutes**

450g/1lb new potatoes, halved if large
450g/1lb green beans, trimmed
1 head round or cos lettuce, torn into bite-size pieces
Two 200g cans tuna in water, drained and broken into large chunks
185g can pitted black olives, drained
2 medium tomatoes, cut into wedges
115g/4oz 95% fat-free Cheddar cheese, cut into 2.5cm/1-inch cubes
8 medium button mushrooms, quartered
115g/4oz pimentos, cut into thin strips
8 tablespoons balsamic vinegar

1. Place the potatoes in a saucepan of boiling water and simmer for about 15 minutes until just tender. Drain and set aside. When cool enough to handle, cut into 2.5cm/1-inch cubes.
2. Meanwhile, boil the green beans for 1 minute. Drain immediately and rinse under cold water to preserve colour.
3. Arrange the salad: divide lettuce among 4 plates and top with even amounts of potatoes, green beans, tuna, olives, tomatoes, cheese, mushrooms and pimentos. Top each serving with 2 tablespoons balsamic vinegar.

nutritional information per serving

calories	protein	carbs	fat	fibre	sodium	cholesterol	calcium
466	17 g	44 g	12 g (23%)	6.5 g	952 mg	46 mg	913 mg

Exercise Must-Do Practice good posture; over the years, poor posture can take a major toll on your back. The very act of standing up straight can balance your body and help maintain the strength of your spine. What's more, you'll look about five pounds lighter than when you slouch.

When standing, tuck in your chin. Keep your back straight and chest held high, shoulders back and relaxed. Keep your stomach and buttock muscles tight. Keep your knees straight but not locked, and your feet parallel.

When sitting, rest your feet flat on the floor, your knees level with your hips. Your middle and lower back should be lightly supported by the back of your chair.

Instant Stress Reliever Let some calming scents take you away from it all. Treat yourself to a bouquet of flowers that includes lavender, and inhale deeply. If you feel tense or agitated, light a vanilla candle or rub on some vanilla-scented body lotion. If stress is distracting you from doing what you need to do, spray a mint, eucalyptus, or citrus body mist for a mental boost.

Daily Weigh-in _____

day 9

Be your own motivator. Buy a new calendar and use it to chronicle your health and fitness progress. Use a blue marker to check off the days when you eat well and a purple marker to mark the days when you exercise. At the end of every week that you see a lot of colour, treat yourself to a small pleasure like a new novel or some make-up. When you don't see a lot of colour, redouble your efforts to eat right and exercise.

Daily Menu

BREAKFAST
1 Slim•Fast Banana Deluxe Powder Shake with ½ banana
   (or your favourite Ultra Slim•Fast shake)
Glass of water

MORNING SNACK
1 Slim•Fast Snack Bar
Glass of water

LUNCH
1 Slim•Fast Ready to Drink Shake
Glass of water

AFTERNOON SNACK
20g/¾oz pretzels
Glass of water

DINNER
Garden Salad

> 55g/2oz mixed greens
> ½ cucumber, peeled and sliced
> 6 cherry tomatoes
> 2 tablespoons fat-free dressing

Beef Fajitas (recipe below)

285g/10oz slice watermelon

Glass of water

EVENING SNACK

15 grapes

Glass of water

day 9 nutritional information

day total	calories	protein	carbs	fat	fibre	sodium	cholesterol	calcium
	1,500	74 g	233 g	30 g (18%)	26 g	1,892 mg	141 mg	1,151 mg

Beef Fajitas

SERVES 4   **total preparation time: 90 minutes**

Marinade

    60ml/2fl oz fresh lime juice

    1 medium jalapeño pepper, finely diced

    1 teaspoon cumin

    2 cloves garlic, crushed

    1 tablespoon vegetable oil

    125ml/4fl oz light beer

780g/1¾ lb joint of beef (topside or silverside)

Vegetable cooking spray

2 medium onions, thinly sliced

2 large green peppers, cored and cut into 5mm/¼-inch strips

2 large tomatoes, diced

4 medium low-fat flour or corn tortillas

55g/2oz salsa

55g/2oz 95% fat-free Cheddar cheese

1. In a shallow dish, mix lime juice, jalapeño pepper, cumin, garlic, vegetable oil and beer. Add beef; cover and place in refrigerator for 20 minutes (or up to 4 hours), turning once.
2. Preheat oven to 220°C/425°F/Gas mark 7.
3. Transfer the beef to a roasting tin and bake 35–45 minutes. Remove to a plate, cover lightly with aluminium foil and let stand for 15–20 minutes (the beef will continue cooking slightly, and will retain its juices). Carve into 5mm/¼-inch-thick slices.
4. Meanwhile, heat a large nonstick frying pan over high heat and coat lightly with vegetable spray. Add onions and peppers and sauté until softened, 3–4 minutes. Add tomatoes and cook 1 minute more, until heated through. Toss well.

5. Spread the tortillas flat on a large plate. Cover one-third of each tortilla with the sautéed vegetables and top with sliced beef, salsa and cheese. Roll the tortilla into a tight wrap and allow to rest 1 minute for the heat of the vegetables to melt the cheese.

nutritional information per serving

	calories	protein	carbs	fat	fibre	sodium	cholesterol	calcium
	555	57 g	42 g	16 g (26%)	3 g	702 mg	126 mg	268 mg

Exercise Must-Do Do this twenty-minute circuit-training workout to tone your shoulders, thighs and arms while giving you a cardio-vascular workout. In between each of these three moves, skip or run on the spot for 30 counts. (You'll need a set of dumbbells, although if you're not very strong you can begin by using full soup cans.)

Shoulder presses Hold a dumbbell in each hand slightly above ear level, with palms facing forward and elbows bent at a 90-degree angle. Straighten arms up until almost fully extended. Return to starting position. Do 15 reps.

Pliés Stand with your feet shoulder-width apart, toes pointing slightly out and knees slightly bent. Hold one dumbbell between legs with both hands and bend your knees until they're at a 90-degree angle, keeping your back straight and your knees in line with your toes. Return to standing position. Do 15 reps.

Biceps curls Stand and hold dumbbells at your sides with palms facing forward. Curl the dumbbells up to chest level, then return to starting position. Do 15 reps.

Instant Stress Reliever Too much to do in too little time? Take a new attitude toward time. Turn your attention away from all the things you have to do, and focus on one thing that's not on your to-do list. Take a moment and really listen to what your children are saying. Try to notice the landscape or interesting buildings when you're driving. Give yourself fifteen minutes a day that are free of interruptions just to be alone with your own thoughts.

Daily Weigh-in _____

day 10

Start keeping a log of how great you feel as you continue to follow the Slim•Fast Plan. When you have a particularly gruelling day (and you feel like you just can't keep up your good health habits), go back and read your log for inspiration.

Daily Menu

BREAKFAST
2 Slim•Fast Meal Replacement Bars
    (or your favourite Ultra Slim•Fast shake)
125ml/4fl oz fresh orange juice
Glass of water

MORNING SNACK
½ bagel (85g/3oz) with 1 tablespoon low-fat soft cheese spread
Glass of water

LUNCH
1 Slim•Fast Chocolate Royale Shake
Glass of water

AFTERNOON SNACK
1 Slim•Fast Snack Bar
Glass of water

DINNER

Spinach Salad

    55g/2oz fresh spinach, chopped

    ½ red onion, sliced

    4 very fresh button mushrooms, sliced

    1 hard-boiled egg, peeled and chopped

    2 tablespoons fat-free dressing

Lemon-Garlic Angel Hair (page 70)

30g/1oz French bread

Fruit Salad

    55g/2oz strawberries

    100g/3½ oz cubed mango (½ medium)

Glass of water

EVENING SNACK

1 pear

Glass of water

day 10 nutritional information

day total	calories	protein	carbs	fat	fibre	sodium	cholesterol	calcium
	1,450	58 g	240 g	28 g (17%)	25 g	1,883 mg	242 mg	1,413 mg

Lemon-Garlic Angel Hair

SERVES 4   total preparation time: **20 minutes**

225g/8oz angel hair pasta
1 tablespoon olive oil
4 cloves garlic, crushed
240ml/8fl oz dry white wine
400g can chopped tomatoes, drained
3 tablespoons lemon juice
Handful fresh basil, chopped or 1 teaspoon dried basil
45g/1½ oz freshly grated Parmesan cheese
¼ teaspoon ground black pepper

1. Bring a large pot of water to the boil over high heat. Add pasta and cook according to package directions until al dente. Drain and place in warm serving bowl.
2. Meanwhile, add olive oil and garlic to a large nonstick frying pan and cook over medium heat for about 30 seconds. Remove pan from heat and pour in white wine. Return pan to medium heat and cook for 1–2 minutes, until wine is reduced by half. Stir in tomatoes, heat for another 1–2 minutes. Remove from the heat, stir in the lemon juice and set aside.
3. Toss the cooked, drained pasta with the basil, Parmesan cheese, black pepper, and tomato mixture.

nutritional information per serving

calories	protein	carbs	fat	fibre	sodium	cholesterol	calcium
322	14 g	40 g	8 g (23%)	3 g	441 mg	10 mg	236 mg

Exercise Must-Do Try this strength-training workout. It doesn't require any specialist equipment – just a sturdy bench or chair.

March on the spot for five-minutes to warm-up. Now do three minutes of bench pushups to work your chest, back, arms and abdominals. Facing a bench or chair, place your hands flat on the seat and walk your feet back until your spine, buttocks and legs are in a straight line and your straightened arms are at a 90-degree angle to the seat. Keeping your abdominal muscles tightened, inhale and bend your arms, lowering yourself down toward the bench. Exhale as you push back up. Aim for 15–20 repetitions. Do two sets, resting for 45 seconds between sets.

Next do some *bench step-ups* for about 3 minutes to work your quadriceps (thighs), hamstrings and buttocks. (If you don't have a bench use the second step on your stairs instead.) Stand facing the bench, with your right foot on the seat. Step straight up with your right leg, touching your left foot briefly on the seat for balance. In a slow, controlled motion, step back down until your left foot is flat on the ground. Immediately do the next step-up with the same leg. Do 10 repetitions and repeat on your left leg. Rest for 45 seconds between each leg. Do 2–3 sets.

Instant Stress Reliever Enjoy some quiet time alone. If the weather is nice, take a walk or bike ride outside. If not, use a treadmill or stationary bike or march on the spot. While you're moving, clear your head of any troubling thoughts and just focus on a thought or word that has personal meaning to you. Keep your mind focused on the movement of your legs, the swinging rhythm of your arms, or the sound of your breath, while letting your mind drift away from any stress or tension.

Daily Weigh-in _____

day 11

Here's a surprising secret: even being a better listener can help your makeover along. Good listening creates greater intimacy in relationships, and can even lower blood pressure in people who have hypertension. Try this listening exercise: sit down with a close friend, family member, or partner for twenty minutes and express how you each feel about whatever is on your minds. Let one person speak for ten minutes, and make sure the listener doesn't respond – even with facial expressions. Next, reverse roles.

Daily Menu

BREAKFAST
1 Slim•Fast Chocolate Royale Ready to Drink Shake
    (or your favourite Ultra Slim•Fast shake)
Glass of water

MORNING SNACK
2 plums
Glass of water

LUNCH
2 Slim•Fast Meal Replacement Bars
Glass of water

AFTERNOON SNACK
115g/4oz fat-free pudding snack
Glass of water

DINNER

Tomato-Cucumber Salad

    1 large tomato, sliced

    1 cucumber, peeled and sliced

    2 tablespoons fat-free dressing

Mediterranean Leg of Lamb with Roasted Vegetables (page 74)

55g/2oz steamed green beans

85g/3oz sugar-free sorbet

Glass of water

EVENING SNACK

1 Slim•Fast Snack Bar

Glass of water

day 11 nutritional information

day total	calories	protein	carbs	fat	fibre	sodium	cholesterol	calcium
	1,465	68 g	219 g	37 g (23%)	24 g	1,118 mg	124 mg	1,109 mg

Mediterranean Leg of Lamb with Roasted Vegetables

SERVES 4   total preparation time: **2 or 2½ hours**

3 cloves garlic

2 teaspoons freshly ground pepper

7g/¼ oz fresh mint, chopped

60ml/2fl oz extra virgin olive oil

2 tablespoons lemon juice

2.25kg/5lb bone-in leg of lamb, trimmed of excess fat

450g/1lb carrots, cut into 5cm/2-inch pieces

4 large onions, cut into quarters

4 medium Désirée or other red potatoes

1. Preheat oven to 230°C/450°F/Gas mark 8.
2. Put the garlic, pepper, mint, olive oil and lemon juice into a food processor. Pulse to blend, about 30 seconds.
3. Place lamb and marinade in large plastic bag and fasten the end. Turn bag over several times, thoroughly rubbing marinade over meat. Refrigerate for 30 minutes, or up to two hours.
4. Remove lamb from plastic bag (discard bag). Place lamb in a large roasting tin with rack. Roast, uncovered, for 15 minutes. Add carrots, onions and potatoes to roasting pan, stirring to coat with lamb juices. Reduce oven temperature to 180°C/350°F/Gas mark 4. Roast for approximately 1½ hours, allowing 15–20 minutes per pound. Remove lamb to serving plate; cover loosely with foil to keep warm. Allow to stand for 15 minutes before serving. Surround lamb with vegetables and serve immediately.

nutritional information per serving

calories	protein	carbs	fat	fibre	sodium	cholesterol	calcium
571	40 g	51 g	24 g (37%)	8 g	133 mg	109 mg	84 mg

Exercise Must-Do Finding it hard to get out of bed in the morning? Feeling that afternoon slump? Squeeze in ten minutes of wake-me-up moves. Dance around for five minutes to your favourite CD, alternating dance moves with knee bends and kicks. Spend the next five minutes doing simple stretches. Stretch #1: Stand straight and fully extend your arms over your head. Try to touch the ceiling; hold for a count of 5. Repeat two more times. Stretch #2: Stand with your feet hip-width apart, knees slightly bent. Bend at your waist to one side as far as is comfortable. Hold for a count of 5. Bring your torso back to centre and repeat, bending to the other side. Do two more repetitions.

Instant Stress Reliever Create an atmosphere that's conducive to a good night's sleep. Use room-darkening shades and ear plugs if traffic is keeping you awake. Sip a cup of camomile tea just before bed. Spray your pillow with some lavender oil, a natural sleep inducer first used by Cleopatra.

Daily Weigh-in _____

day 12

If you're always expending energy to keep yourself together, looking good and acting the way you feel you're supposed to, you may wish you could just be yourself for a while. Letting go this way can lead to heightened creativity, honesty and more genuine contact with other people – and yourself.

Daily Menu

BREAKFAST

1 Slim•Fast French Vanilla Powder Shake
    (or your favourite Ultra Slim•Fast shake)
Glass of water

MORNING SNACK

1 Slim•Fast Snack Bar
Glass of water

LUNCH

1 Slim•Fast Ready to Drink Shake
Glass of water

AFTERNOON SNACK

115g/4oz very low fat cottage cheese with 85g/3oz diced peaches
    (fresh or canned)
Glass of water

DINNER

Tossed Salad

  55g/2oz mixed greens

  1 small red onion, sliced

  85g/3oz beetroot

  2 tablespoons fat-free dressing

Salmon Supreme (page 78)

55g/2oz steamed peas

115g/4oz steamed summer squash

1 kiwi fruit, sliced

Glass of water

EVENING SNACK

¼ cantaloupe melon

Glass of water

day 12 nutritional information

day total	calories	protein	carbs	fat	fibre	sodium	cholesterol	calcium
	1,429	95 g	215 g	24 g (15%)	33 g	1,778 mg	142 mg	1,300 mg

Salmon Supreme

SERVES 4   total preparation time: **25 minutes**

Vegetable cooking spray

4 medium Désirée or other red potatoes, washed and cut into 5mm/¼-inch slices

Four 200g/7oz salmon steaks, about 2.5cm/1 inch thick

2 tablespoons lemon juice

2 tablespoons virtually fat-free fromage frais

55g/2oz 90% fat-free mayonnaise-style dressing

¼ teaspoon ground black pepper

2 large carrots, grated

2 medium tomatoes, finely diced

1 spring onion, finely diced

½ lemon, cut into 4 wedges

1. Preheat oven to 200°C/400°F/Gas mark 6. Spray a medium roasting tin with vegetable spray.
2. Rinse salmon and pat dry. Place potatoes and salmon in a single layer in roasting tin and drizzle fish with 1 tablespoon lemon juice.
3. In a small bowl, combine remaining tablespoon lemon juice with fromage frais, mayonnaise and pepper, and mix until smooth. Stir in carrots, tomatoes and spring onion. Top fish and potatoes with vegetable mixture, spreading on top of all.
4. Bake, uncovered, until potatoes are tender and fish flakes easily, 12 minutes. Preheat grill. Place under grill for 60 seconds to brown vegetable mixture. Serve immediately. Garnish with lemon wedges.

nutritional information per serving

	calories	protein	carbs	fat		fibre	sodium	cholesterol	calcium
	465	45 g	39 g	14 g (27%)		4.5 g	258 mg	112 mg	65 mg

Exercise Must-Do Increase your balance and control with this exercise. Stand with your feet flat directly under your hips, your hands on your hips and your abdominal muscles contracted. Bend your right knee, lifting your leg in front of you until your right heel is level with your left knee. With your left hand, press on your right inner thigh, resisting with the muscle. Put your hands back on your hips. Next, keeping hips and shoulders pointing straight ahead and your right foot resting gently on the inside of your left knee, squeeze the muscles in your left leg and pivot your right knee out to the side. Hold for a second, return your knee to the forward-facing position, and lower your foot to the ground. Do 10 reps, alternating sides.

Instant Stress Reliever Practice mindfulness – a heightened state of alertness that will put you more in touch with the world around you. Notice a pen's shape, colour, weight and feel. Sip a cup of warm peppermint tea, focusing on the heat of the liquid and the smell of the mint. Savour a single strawberry and feel its juices wet your tongue. Mindfulness leads to relaxation.

Daily Weigh-in _____

day 13

Don't shy away from taking on a project with a heavy workload because you think it will make you stressed and unhappy. People who work long hours because they're trying to achieve a goal they've set for themselves – as opposed to working under extreme pressure from above – are usually happy about the work they're doing. So pursue your lofty goals, and look forward to your accomplishments!

Daily Menu

BREAKFAST

1 Slim•Fast Chocolate Royale Powder Shake
    (or your favourite Ultra Slim•Fast shake)
Glass of water

MORNING SNACK

115g/4oz canned fruit (snack pack)
Glass of water

LUNCH

1 Slim•Fast Ready to Drink Shake
15 baby carrots
Glass of water

AFTERNOON SNACK

1 Slim•Fast Snack Bar
Glass of water

DINNER

Black Bean Salad

130g/4½ oz canned black beans, drained

55g/2oz diced red pepper

30g/1oz diced onion

2 tablespoons balsamic vinegar

6 lettuce leaves

Chicken Stir-Fry with White Rice (page 82)

85g/3oz canned pineapple chunks in juice

Glass of water

EVENING SNACK

85g/3oz air-popped popcorn

Glass of water

day 13 nutritional information

day total	calories	protein	carbs	fat	fibre	sodium	cholesterol	calcium
	1,507	85 g	244 g	27 g (16%)	40 g	1,426 mg	130 mg	982 mg

Chicken Stir-Fry with White Rice

SERVES 4   **total preparation time: 40 minutes**

200g/7oz long-grain white rice

1 tablespoon olive oil

3 cloves garlic, crushed

780g/1¾ lb boneless chicken breasts, sliced into strips

1 tablespoon light (reduced-sodium) soy sauce

60ml/2fl oz low-sodium chicken stock

1 teaspoon ground ginger

½ teaspoon celery seed

450g/1lb broccoli, cut into florets

450g/1lb carrots, cut into 1cm/½-inch slices

450g/1lb mushrooms, sliced

1 medium green pepper, cored and cut into strips

1 medium red pepper, cored and cut into strips

1. In a medium saucepan, combine rice with 500ml/18fl oz water and bring to the boil. Immediately reduce heat to very low, cover and simmer 20 minutes. Take it off the heat and allow it to sit 5–10 minutes; fluff with a fork before serving.

2. While the rice is cooking, heat the oil in a wok or large frying pan over medium-high heat. Sauté garlic until golden, 30–60 seconds. Add chicken and sauté, turning frequently, 5–7 minutes or until cooked through. Remove chicken from pan and set aside.

3. In a small bowl, mix soy sauce, stock, ginger, celery seed and vegetables. Sauté in the same pan over medium heat until vegetables are slightly softened but still crisp, 3–4 minutes. Return chicken to mixture and mix well. Serve immediately with the hot white rice.

nutritional information per serving

	calories	protein	carbs	fat		fibre	sodium	cholesterol	calcium
	598	52 g	61 g	16 g (24%)		8 g	327 mg	120 mg	117 mg

Exercise Must-Do Maximize your walking technique to help you burn more calories without burning yourself out.

- While walking, keep your eyes focused on a spot a few metres in front of you instead of looking at the ground.
- Clench your hands into loose fists and swing them without crossing them (which would twist your torso and slow you down).
- Maintain a short, quick, efficient stride by letting your foot land practically beneath you. Don't step out, but keep more of your stride length behind your body, not in front of it.
- Keep your back straight; neck and shoulders relaxed.
- To soften your landing, try to touch the ground heel first with your ankle flexed, then roll forward to the front of your foot. Push off with flexed toes for your next step.

Instant Stress Reliever The Chinese have developed a series of exercises that promote the flow of chi, the life force that flows through the body and regulates its functions.

- Stand with your feet shoulder-width apart and parallel. Bend your knees to a quarter-squat position (about 45 degrees) while keeping your upper body straight. Observe your breathing for a couple of breaths.
- Inhale and bring your arms slowly up in front of you to shoulder height with your elbows slightly bent. Exhale, stretching your arms straight out.
- Inhale again, bend your elbows slightly and slowly drop your arms down until your thumbs touch the sides of your legs.
- Exhale one more time, then stand up straight.

Daily Weigh-in _____

day 14

Devise a daily affirmation that will help you stay your course on the weight-loss track for life. The next time you're feeling tempted to over indulge, repeat ten times, 'I am healthy, I am strong. I am doing what's best for me.'

Daily Menu

BREAKFAST
2 Slim•Fast Meal Replacement Bars
125ml/4fl oz cranberry juice
Glass of water

MORNING SNACK
225g/8oz virtually fat-free fruit yogurt, artificially sweetened
Glass of water

LUNCH
1 Slim•Fast Strawberry Supreme Powder Shake
Glass of water

AFTERNOON SNACK
Vegetable Sticks

    1 red pepper, cored and cut into strips

    1 celery stick, cut into strips

    1 tablespoon very low fat cottage cheese

Glass of water

DINNER

Garden Salad (page 86)

Split Pea Soup (page 87)

Herbed Whole-Grain Bread (page 88)

⅛ honeydew melon

Glass of water

EVENING SNACK

1 Slim•Fast Snack Bar

Glass of water

day 14 nutritional information

day total	calories	protein	carbs	fat	fibre	sodium	cholesterol	calcium
	1,422	70 g	248 g	21 g (13%)	33 g	1,174 mg	30 mg	1,375 mg

Garden Salad

total preparation time: **12 minutes**

1 small head red-leaf lettuce, torn into bite-size pieces

1 small head cos lettuce, torn into bite-size pieces

1 large cucumber, peeled and thinly sliced

8 radishes, thinly sliced

24 cherry tomatoes, halved

125ml/4fl oz fat-free dressing

In a large salad bowl, toss all ingredients except dressing. Dress immediately before serving.

nutritional information per serving

calories	protein	carbs	fat	fibre	sodium	cholesterol	calcium
74	3 g	16 g	1 g (10%)	4 g	37 mg	0 mg	56 mg

Split Pea Soup

SERVES 4   total preparation time: **1 hour 10minutes**

450g/1lb dried yellow or green split peas
2 teaspoons olive oil
3 cloves garlic, crushed
1.2 litres/40fl oz chicken or vegetable stock
250ml/8fl oz water

1. Rinse the split peas, drain and set aside.
2. Place olive oil in a large saucepan over medium-high heat. Add garlic and sauté until golden, 30 seconds. Add split peas, stock and water, increase heat to high and bring to the boil. Reduce heat to low, cover and simmer until peas are tender when mashed, 45 minutes.

nutritional information per serving

calories	protein	carbs	fat	fibre	sodium	cholesterol	calcium
447	31 g	73 g	5 g (11%)	16 g	180 mg	5 mg	69 mg

Herbed Whole-Grain Bread

SERVES 4   total preparation time: **5 minutes**

4 teaspoons diet margarine
4 thick slices whole-grain bread
¼ teaspoon garlic powder
½ teaspoon poppy seeds
½ teaspoon chives (or substitute your favourite herb)

1. Preheat grill.
2. Spread a thin layer of margarine on bread and sprinkle with garlic powder, poppy seeds and chives. Grill close to the heat until edges are golden, 30–60 seconds.

nutritional information per serving

calories	protein	carbs	fat	fibre	sodium	cholesterol	calcium
94	3 g	14 g	3 g (29%)	1 g	187 mg	0 mg	37 mg

Exercise Must-Do Whether you choose to take a walk or go for a bike ride, try exercising with a partner. You can be each other's personal trainer and motivate each other to push harder. Choose a friend, your spouse, or even your dog. No matter who you're with, you'll see that working out in tandem drives away boredom and makes exercise fun!

Instant Stress Reliever To get into a relaxed state of being, apply some acupressure, which stimulates the same pressure points as acupuncture but uses fingers instead of needles. Find the 'Third Eye', located between the eyebrows, in the indentation where the bridge of the nose meets the forehead. Breathe deeply and apply firm, steady pressure on each point for two to three minutes. The pressure should cause a mild aching sensation, but not pain.

Your First Steps to Success

Congratulations: you've completed the 14-Day Plan. You've dedicated two weeks to your own fitness and health, and you've probably already begun to feel the results. Have you felt more relaxed? More energetic? Happier? Terrific. You've probably lost a few pounds – and even if it's only a start, at least you've seen that you can do it. You've seen that living healthy doesn't mean living a lifestyle of restrictions, deprivations, or denials.

So where do we go from here?

The following chapters discuss the basics of nutrition and exercise: why they're important for your health, and how you can work good health habits into your life – on your own terms. The 14-Day Plan gave you a sense of how good a new lifestyle can make you feel. But you can't stay on a prescribed plan forever. It's time to help you tailor a plan that fits comfortably into your life. It's time for you to create your own full-time makeover.

5

balanced nutrition for a healthy life

Now that you've begun to learn just how good you can feel on the road to weight loss and fitness, it is time to incorporate these changes into your everyday life. Before you get started, however, it's important to understand some basics about nutrition – the process that keeps your body working efficiently. In the past quarter-century, myths about nutrition have flown thick and fast, each one more alarming and irresistible than the last. We've been told we need to avoid all fat; that we should ban red meat from our diet; that we can eat as much of a food as we like – as long as it's a fat-free product. Wrong, wrong, wrong – and in this chapter you'll see why.

The truth is, trying to understand nutrition can be confusing, even discouraging – especially with the constant parade of new studies we're always hearing about in the news. Remember when fat became a nutritional villain, until it was suddenly dubbed an essential part of our diets. It's like the scene in the movie *Sleeper* where Woody Allen goes into the future, only to discover that organic rice has been deemed unhealthy and that cigarette smoking can actually help you live longer.

What you may find surprising is that the basic definition of good nutrition hasn't really changed much in the past thirty years. It's still important to eat lots of fruits and vegetables, eat fat in moderation and eat plenty of unrefined complex carbohydrates such as oatmeal, brown rice and wholemeal bread. Consuming a variety of foods is still the best way to give your body a balanced supply of nutrients. If you hear that your favourite vegetable can help prevent cancer, it's fine to include a few extra servings in your diet each week. What you shouldn't do is load up on that one particular vegetable and forgo the rest.

Nutritional researchers know they'll never find one magic food that will keep our bodies healthy and prevent disease. That's why they recommend aiming for a rainbow diet that includes as many colours of fruits and vegetables as you can possibly get. The chemicals that put the purple in plums, the red in tomatoes and the green in spinach – phytochemicals, as they're called – can help combat disease by neutralizing cancer-causing substances lurking within the body. Eating lots of produce will also help you get a wide variety of vitamins, including antioxidants that have been shown to help fight disease.

This is just one aspect of good nutrition. Another involves the kind of sensible advice your grandmother gave you: eat all foods in moderation. The fact is, you don't need to banish any foods as long as you eat a nutritionally balanced diet. As you read on, you may be surprised to learn that you've been going overboard to avoid certain foods – and excited to find that making a small change in your diet can help improve your health and take off those stubborn pounds.

The Truth About Fat

Fat makes you fat; avoid it at all costs. You've probably recited similar words in your head time and time again. After all, high-fat foods *are* a concentrated source of calories, and when consumed in excess they can lead to obesity and raise your risk of heart disease and certain cancers. And carbohydrates and protein (which contain 4 calories per gram) have less than half the calories of fat (9 calories per gram).

So, isn't it better to avoid fat altogether? No, say experts. Just because a low-fat diet is good for you doesn't mean a no-fat diet is better. What's important is to watch your fat intake and not let it creep above the recommended level – something that's easy to do on the Slim•Fast Plan.

Health experts recommend you should get no more than 30 per cent of your total calories from fat, although a significant number believe the figure should be closer to 20–25 per cent. Others contend that if your diet is high in monounsaturated fats, you don't have to worry about going over the 30 per cent mark.

Following the Slim•Fast Makeover, you'll get about 20 per cent of your total calories from fat, a low level that should help you lose weight and improve your health. At 1,400–1,500 calories per day (the weight-loss plan's allotment), you should be eating about 31 grams of fat each day. A Slim•Fast shake contains no more than 3 grams of fat, so the bulk of the fat in your diet will come from your meals and snacks. Although you should read labels for the fat content, you shouldn't make fat grams the sole determining factor in your diet. Simply choose foods that are naturally low in saturated fat and use olive, rapeseed and peanut oils, which are rich in monounsaturated fats.

Use the following chart as a guide to making wise food choices:

INSTEAD OF...	CHOOSE...
semi-skimmed milk	skimmed milk
(240ml/8fl oz: 118 cal, 4 g fat)	(240ml/8fl oz: 82 cal, 0.3 g fat)
corn oil	olive oil
(1 tablespoon: 120 cal;	(1 tablespoon: 120 cal;
2 g saturated fat,	2 g saturated fat,
8 g polyunsaturated fat,	1 g polyunsaturated fat,
4 g monounsaturated fat)	10 g monounsaturated fat)
dark meat chicken	white meat chicken
(thigh, drumstick with skin)	(breast, skinless)
(170g/6oz: 430 cal, 27 g fat)	(170g/6oz: 281 cal, 6 g fat)
Cheddar cheese	reduced-fat Cheddar cheese
(55g/2oz: 229 cal, 19 g fat)	(55g/2oz: 162 cal, 9 g fat)
croissant	oat bran bagel
(85g/3oz: 345 cal, 18 g fat)	(85g/3oz: 217 cal, 1 g fat)
doughnut	Garibaldi biscuits
(55g/2oz: 239 cal, 13 g fat)	(55g/2oz: 204 cal, 6 g fat)

The Lowdown on Carbohydrates

In the early 1990s, we were in the midst of a love affair with carbohydrates. Pasta and bread were seen as freebies – since they had little fat, many thought they'd be a great way to help lose weight. We let portions go to the wind – and we watched ourselves get fatter, not thinner. The failure of these high-carb diets caused the pendulum to swing the other way. Suddenly carbohydrates were the culprits behind every health ill from diabetes to heart disease to obesity. Now high-protein diets are the latest fad, as we struggle to divorce ourselves from starchy foods.

Like any food hailed as a panacea, carbohydrates have toppled off their high pedestal. After all, they do contain calories, and enough of those calories can make you fat. That said, the carbohydrate equation becomes a bit more complicated. A huge variety of foods fall into the carb category: fruits, vegetables and sugar are the simple carbs, and pasta, bread, potatoes and other starches are complex carbs. Simple or complex, your body breaks down all the carbohydrates into a single sugar called glucose, which is used for fuel. That's about where the similarities between the different types of carbs end.

Nutritionally, all carbohydrates are not created equal. A high-fibre, low-sugar carb (a peach, for instance) is a lot less calorie-dense than a low-fibre, high-sugar carb (a piece of peach pie). Your body breaks down low-fibre, highly processed carbs much faster, which is why you get a quick energy boost after eating sweetened cereal or a glass of juice. Your body breaks down unrefined, high-fibre carbs (fresh fruits and vegetables, wholemeal bread and rice, oatmeal) more gradually, which gives you a steadier stream of energy and helps you feel sated.

For many of us refined sugar – usually in the context of biscuits, cakes and other snack foods – is the carb we eat most. Refined sugar intake has been rising steadily over the years but one often-overlooked culprit is the reduced-fat treats that are full of sugar instead of fat. Unfortunately, extra sugar means extra calories. In fact, many reduced-fat and fat-free products contain nearly as many calories as their full-fat counterparts. Of course, it's fine to replace your regular biscuits or ice-cream with reduced-fat versions – just don't give yourself licence to eat more. Stick with the serving-size portion, and remember that if you go overboard you can easily eat far more calories than you normally would.

Keep in mind, too, that *sugar is not a bad food that deserves to be banned* from your diet. Foods with a lot of refined sugar, however, usually contain little nutrition and a lot of calories. Your best bet is to save the sugary sweets for special occasions. On the other hand, the little sugar packet on the table that you use to flavour your coffee won't destroy your diet. If you prefer sugar to saccharine or aspartame, allow yourself a little of the real thing. It has only 16 calories per teaspoon. Just use it sparingly.

Of much more nutritional value are the carbs that are high in fibre, an indigestible form of carbohydrate found only in plants. Eating fibre-rich foods can make you feel fuller for longer, lower your cholesterol, and provide the bulk necessary to promote regularity and prevent constipation. What's more, the higher the dietary fibre in a food, the less fat and calories it contains and the more slowly it's absorbed by the body.

Since fibre slows digestion, you feel fuller between meals – which can actually help you eat less at the next meal. A study from the International Life Sciences Institute found that eating high-fibre foods for breakfast or lunch appears to reduce food intake at the next meal. At up to 5 grams per serving, Slim•Fast shakes are a good source of fibre. Here are some other high-fibre stars, any of which you can include in your personal eating plan:

FOOD	SERVING SIZE	MODERATE FIBRE (2–4 G)	HIGH FIBRE (5+ G)
Breads	1 slice	wholemeal, cracked wheat	
	4	rye wafers	
Cereals	30g/1oz	Bran Flakes, Raisin Bran, Shredded Wheat, oatmeal	All Bran
Vegetables	55g/2oz	beetroot, broccoli, Brussels sprouts, cabbage, carrots, corn, green beans, green peas, frozen spinach (boiled)	
	1 medium	baked potato with skin	corn on the cob
Fruits	1 medium	apple with peel, date, fig, mango, nectarine, orange, pear, banana	
	55g/2oz	apple sauce (unsweetened), raspberries, blackberries	cooked prunes
Legumes	85g/3oz	kidney beans, black beans, chickpeas, lentils, broad beans, baked beans	

How Much Protein Do You Really Need?

High-protein diets have recently grown in popularity, billing themselves as the final answer to the obesity question. The truth is, you can lose weight on a high-protein diet the same as you can on any other diet. The real trouble is that these diets don't have much staying power. After a while, we get sick of eating meat, chicken and fish for breakfast, lunch and dinner, and begin to crave the bread that's missing from our sandwiches and the crisps that are banned as snacks.

What's more, many nutritionists frown on high-protein diets

because they don't provide you with the balanced nutrition your body needs. The Slim•Fast Makeover will give you the proper balance of protein, carbs, and fat – based on the sensible guidelines of the U.S. Department of Agriculture. On the Makeover, you'll be getting about 20 per cent of your calories from fat, 55 per cent from carbohydrates and 25 per cent from protein. The Slim•Fast eating plan calls for you to consume about 88 grams of protein a day. Two Slim•Fast shakes plus one 170g/6oz serving of meat, chicken, fish, or vegetable protein should fulfil your protein requirement.

Protein is an essential nutrient that is the basis of all life; after water, it's the most plentiful substance in the human body, composing most of your muscle mass, skin, hair, eyes and nails. And the real secret to having sustained energy throughout the day lies in eating the right combination of protein and carbohydrates – which you'll find on the Slim•Fast Makeover. Carbs will cause an immediate rise in your blood sugar, protein will boost it later, and your energy levels will be sustained until your next meal. The goal to aim for is one gram of high-quality protein for every pound of your goal body weight.

What's high-quality protein? Just as with carbohydrates and fats, the key to protein lies in choosing the right kinds. Many traditional sources of protein – red meat and dairy produce in particular – are now available in reduced fat options, whether it is a leaner cut of meat or a low-fat alternative to cream. You can also choose reduced-fat cheese and yogurt. These are packed with protein with little or no saturated fat or cholesterol.

Protein from plant sources – grains, vegetables, legumes, soya, nuts and seeds – packs an even larger nutritional punch. They contain virtually no fat and are loaded with phytochemicals that can help ward off disease. By replacing some of your animal protein consumption with plant proteins, you'll be doing yourself a favour. Some rich plant-protein foods include cooked soya beans, tofu, kidney beans, bulgur wheat and oatmeal.

Calcium: Are You Getting Enough?

A surprisingly large number of women don't get enough calcium, which is thought to help protect against osteoporosis later in life. This is because many calcium-rich foods like cheese and ice-cream also tend to be high in fat and calories. So if you're trying to lose weight, you're probably also trying to avoid these foods.

Long hailed as the best bone-builder around, calcium has an amazing host of other health benefits. In a recent study, researchers tested the effects of three eating plans to see which one was most effective at preventing hypertension: standard Western fare (high in animal protein and refined carbohydrates) was compared against a diet high in fruits and vegetables and a combination diet that was rich in fruits, vegetables and low-fat dairy products (similar to the Slim●Fast eating plan). The study found that the combination diet was as effective at controlling high blood pressure as some antihypertensive medications, while the diet without the low-fat dairy allotment was only about half as effective. Calcium is believed to reduce blood pressure by causing the production of a chemical that causes blood vessels to relax and open up. Other research suggests that a diet rich in calcium may help ease premenstrual syndrome. Scientific evidence also finds that high-calcium foods pack more punch than supplements. You should get 1,000 mg of calcium daily; here's a list of ten top calcium-rich foods:

FOOD	SERVING	CALCIUM (MG)	CALORIES	FAT (GRAMS)
Skimmed milk	250ml/8fl oz	301	82	Less than 1
Yogurt, natural, very low fat	225g/8oz	487	90	Less than 1
Slim•Fast Ready-to-Drink shake	325ml can	400	220	3
Tofu (processed with calcium sulfate)	115g/4oz	397	86	5
Calcium-fortified orange juice	250ml/8fl oz	350	110	0
Salmon, canned, drained with bones	85g/3oz	203	130	6
Orange	1 medium	52	62	0
Broccoli, boiled, drained	55g/2oz	36	22	Less than 1
Cos lettuce	100g/3½oz	40	16	0
Cottage cheese, 1% milkfat	115g/4oz	99	79	1

The Key Vitamins and Minerals You Need

Vitamins and minerals are key nutrients your body uses to help the normal functioning of cells. They can help promote good vision, form normal blood cells, create strong bones and teeth, and ensure the proper functioning of the heart and brain. There are thirteen vitamins we need most: vitamins A, C, D, E, K, and eight B-complex vitamins – thiamine, riboflavin, niacin, B6, pantothenic acid, biotin, folic acid and B12. Each of these vitamins carries out specific functions and if a certain vitamin isn't supplied through our diet over a long period of time, a particular deficiency disease usually results.

Like vitamins, minerals are also essential for your body to perform a host of vital functions, from basic bone formation to the regulation of your heartbeat to the normal functioning of digestion. Although there are sixty different types of minerals in your body, only twenty-two essential minerals are necessary for your diet. These include large or macro-minerals, including calcium, magnesium, phosphorus, potassium and sodium, and small or micro-minerals such as chromium, copper, iron, manganese, molybdenum, selenium and zinc.

Since vitamins and minerals can ward off certain diseases caused by deficiencies, you might assume that the more, the better. But science says otherwise. The bulk of the vitamin research studies indicate that vitamins and minerals don't bestow additional health benefits if taken in amounts much greater than the recommended daily allowance (RDA). In fact, some vitamins (like vitamins A and D) can be toxic if taken in excessive amounts.

Unless your doctor advises you to take a certain supplement, you can meet your vitamin and mineral needs by drinking two Slim•Fast shakes a day – which are fortified with up to twenty-four essential vitamins and minerals – along with a variety of fruits and vegetables and a balanced meal. Each milk-based shake gives you more than a third of the RDA for most vitamins and minerals, including calcium, vitamin E and vitamin C. You should have no trouble getting the rest of the vitamins and minerals you need from the foods you eat. The following two charts contain a quick rundown of the essential vitamins and minerals – which foods to get them from and how your body uses them.

Vitamins: Where to Get Them, How You Use Them

VITAMIN	FOOD SOURCE	WHAT IT DOES
Vitamin A	Liver, eggs, fortified milk, carrots, tomatoes, apricots, cantaloupe melon, fish	Promotes good vision, helps form and maintain healthy skin and mucous membranes; may protect against some cancers
Vitamin C	Citrus fruits, strawberries, tomatoes	Promotes healthy gums, capillaries and teeth; aids iron absorption; may block production of nitrosamines; maintains normal connective tissue; aids in healing wounds
Vitamin D	Fortified milk, fish; also produced by the body in in response to sunlight	Promotes strong bones and teeth; necessary for absorption of calcium
Vitamin E	Nuts, vegetable oils, whole grains, olives, asparagus, spinach	Protects tissue against damage from cancer-causing substances; important in formation of red blood cells; helps body use vitamin K. May prevent or alleviate coronary heart disease
Vitamin K	Body produces about half of daily needs; cauliflower, broccoli, cabbage, spinach, cereals, soya beans, beef liver	Aids in clotting of blood
Vitamin B1 (thiamine)	Whole grains, dried beans, lean meats (especially pork), fish	Helps release energy from carbohydrates; necessary for healthy brain and nerve cells and for functioning of heart

Vitamin B2 (riboflavin)	Nuts, dairy products, liver	Aids in release of energy from foods; interacts with other B vitamins
Vitamin B3 (niacin)	Nuts, dairy products, liver	Aids in release of energy from foods; involved in synthesis of DNA; maintains normal functioning of skin, nerves, and digestive system
Vitamin B5 (pantothenic acid)	Whole grains, dried beans, eggs, nuts	Aids in the release of energy from foods; essential for synthesis of numerous body materials
Vitamin B6 (pyridoxine)	Whole grains, dried beans, eggs, nuts	Important in chemical reactions of proteins and amino acids; involved in normal functioning of brain and formation of red blood cells
Vitamin B12	Liver, beef, eggs, milk, shellfish	Necessary for development of red blood cells; maintains normal functioning of nervous system
Folic acid	Liver, wheat bran, leafy green vegetables, beans, grains	Important in synthesis of DNA; acts together with B12 in the production of haemoglobin (which carries oxygen through the blood)
Biotin	Yeast, eggs, liver, milk	Important in formation of fatty acids; helps metabolize amino acids and carbohydrates

Source: University of California Berkeley, *The Wellness Encyclopedia* (Houghton Mifflin, 1991).

Minerals: Where to Get Them, How You Use Them

MINERAL	FOOD SOURCE	WHAT IT DOES
Calcium	Milk and milk products, sardines and salmon eaten with bone, dark green leafy vegetables, shellfish, hard water	Builds bones and teeth, maintains bone density and strength; helps prevent osteoporosis; helps regulate heartbeat, blood clotting, muscle contraction and nerve conduction
Chloride	Table salt, fish	Maintains normal fluid shifts; balances blood pH; forms stomach acid to aid in digestion
Magnesium	Wheat bran, whole grains, raw leafy green vegetables, nuts (especially almonds and cashews), soya beans, bananas, apricots, spices	Aids in bone growth; aids function of nerves and muscle, including regulation of normal heart rhythm
Phosphorus	Meats, poultry, fish, cheese, egg yolks, dried peas and beans, milk and milk products, soft drinks, nuts; present in almost all foods	Aids in bone growth and strengthening of teeth; important in energy metabolism
Potassium	Oranges and orange juice, bananas, dried fruits, peanut butter, dried peas and beans, potatoes, coffee, tea, cocoa, yogurt, molasses, meat	Promotes regular heartbeat; active in muscle contraction; regulates transfer of nutrients to cells; controls water balance in body tissues and cells; helps regulate blood pressure

Sodium	Table salt, salt added to prepared foods, baking soda	Helps regulate water balance in body; plays a role in maintaining blood pressure
Chromium	Meat, cheese, whole grains, dried peas and beans, peanuts	Important for glucose metabolism; may be a cofactor for insulin
Copper	Shellfish, nuts, beef and pork liver, cocoa powder, chocolate, kidneys, dried beans, raisins, corn oil margarine	Formation of red blood cells; cofactor in absorbing iron into blood cells; helps produce several respiratory enzymes
Fluorine (fluoride)	Fluoridated water and foods grown or cooked in it; fish, tea, gelatine	Contributes to solid bone and tooth formation; may help prevent osteoporosis
Iodine	Primarily from iodized salt, but also seafood, seaweed food products, vegetables grown in iodine-rich areas, vegetable oil	Necessary for normal function of the thyroid gland and for normal cell function; keeps skin, hair and nails healthy; prevents goiter
Iron	Liver, kidneys, red meats, egg yolks, peas, beans, nuts, dried fruits, green leafy vegetables, enriched grain products	Essential to formation of haemoglobin (which carries oxygen through the blood); part of several enzymes and proteins in the body
Manganese	Nuts, whole grains, vegetables, fruits, instant coffee, tea, cocoa powder, beetroot, egg yolks	Required for normal bone growth and development, normal reproduction and cell function
Molybdenum	Peas, beans, cereal grains, organ meats, some dark green vegetables	Important for normal cell function

| Selenium | Fish, shellfish, red meat, egg yolks, chicken, garlic, tuna, tomatoes | Complements vitamin E to fight cell damage by certain cancer-causing substances called free radicals |
| Zinc | Oysters, crabmeat, beef, liver, eggs, poultry, brewer's yeast, wholemeal bread | Maintains taste and smell acuity; normal growth and sexual development; important for fetal growth and wound healing |

Source: University of California, Berkeley, *The Wellness Encyclopedia* (Houghton Mifflin, 1991).

Water: The Forgotten Nutrient

You must have heard it numerous times before: drink two litres (3½ pints) of water a day to stay healthy. A vital nutrient that makes up 55–60 per cent of your body weight, water stabilizes body temperature, carries nutrients to and waste away from cells, and is needed for cells to function. Water also aids in digestion and helps prevent constipation, and it works wonders at filling you up when you drink it with a meal.

Now, let's be honest. Do you actually make a concerted effort to drink what amounts to about eight 250ml/8fl oz glasses of fluid each day, plus another three or four after you've been out in the heat or exercising? Or, like most of us, do you just take a drink when you feel thirsty?

Unfortunately, judging by your own feeling of thirst may not be enough: often we don't feel thirsty until our bodies reach a dehydration danger point. You may lose up to two litres of water before thirst prompts you to start drinking. In general, feeling thirsty means dehydration is setting in.

Not drinking enough water can be damaging to your health. Getting dehydrated during a workout can lead to premature fatigue and raises your risk of heat exhaustion and heatstroke on a hot day. Dehydration can cause fatigue and make you feel headachy, dizzy and nauseated. And not drinking enough water on a day-to-day basis can leave you feeling out of sorts. However, drinking dehydrating beverages such as coffee, tea, caffeinated soft drinks and alcohol does *not* make up the shortfall. Alcohol and caffeine are diuretics, substances that cause the body to lose water through urination.

Fortunately, you shouldn't have much difficulty getting the water you need if you follow these basic rules of thumb:

- **Get the equivalent of 8 glasses of water a day.** If you drink coffee, alcohol, or other dehydrating beverages, offset the loss of water by drinking an additional glass of water for every dehydrating beverage you drink. This means 10 glasses of water a day if you have a cup of coffee or tea in the morning and a diet cola with lunch.
- **Drink before you exercise, as well as during and afterward.** Ideally, you should drink two 250ml/8fl oz cups of water two hours before your activity. You'll lose any excess through urination before you begin to exercise. If you can't drink water two hours in advance, have a 250ml/8fl oz glass just before you begin. While you're exercising, drink 180–340ml/6–12fl oz of water every fifteen to twenty minutes, especially when you're outdoors in the heat.
- **Use your weight as a guide.** Weigh yourself before and after your workout – preferably unclothed, since sweaty clothes weigh more than dry ones. For each pound less that you weigh after your workout, drink about 500ml/18fl oz of water to replace the water you lost as sweat.
- **Keep a large bottle of water nearby.** Place it on your desk at work or on the kitchen table. You'll be reminded to drink throughout the day and you may find it helps control your hunger. What you think is hunger may really be a craving for water.

Foods That Prevent Disease

Even in this technological day and age, scientists would be hard pressed to create the perfect food – a food that contains all the nutrients that your body needs. Slim•Fast and other meal replacement products contain nutrients such as fat, protein and carbohydrates as well as fibre and a host of essential vitamins and minerals. But they don't contain the hundreds of other hidden nutrients that scientists continue to learn more about every day. These are tiny molecules called phytochemicals that act almost like medicine to impart health benefits beyond basic nutrition. Some phytochemicals reduce your risk of cancer or heart disease; others prevent gastrointestinal problems. All can help you stay healthy, and you won't find most of them in a pill. The fact is, scientists still don't know how all the phytochemicals work.

How can you get a dose of this medicine? Eat a variety of fruits and vegetables to get a variety of phytochemicals. Here are just a few of the key phytochemicals you need:

Examples of Foods That Can Prevent Disease

TYPE OF PHYTOCHEMICAL	SOURCE	POTENTIAL BENEFIT
Antiadhesion component (not fully identified)	Cranberry juice	May improve urinary tract health
Carotenoids		
Alpha-carotene	Carrots	Neutralize free radicals that
Beta-carotene	Fruits, vegetables	may cause damage to cells, turning a normal cell into a cancerous one
Lutein	Green vegetables	
Lycopene	Tomato products (sauces etc.)	

Zeaxanthin	Eggs, citrus, corn	
Dietary Fibre		
Insoluble fibre	Wheat bran, vegetables	May reduce risk of breast or colon cancer
Soluble fibre	Oats, barley, fruits	Reduce risk of cardiovascular disease
Flavonoids		
Anthocyanidins	Fruits	Neutralize free radicals,
Catechins	Tea	may reduce risk of cancer
Flavanones	Citrus	
Flavones	Fruits/vegetables	
Glucosinolates, indoles, isothiocyanates sulphoraphane	Cruciferous vegetables (broccoli, kale, horseradish)	Neutralize free radicals, stimulate anti-cancer enzymes
Phenols		
Caffeic acid	Fruits,	Antioxidant-like activities may
Ferulic acid	vegetables, citrus	reduce risk of degenerative diseases, heart disease, eye disease
Phytoestrogens		
Isoflavones		
Diadzein	Soya beans and	May protect against heart
Genistein	soya-based foods	disease and some cancers; may lower LDL cholesterol
Lignans	Flax, rye, vegetables	
Prebiotics/probiotics		
Lactobacillus	Yogurt, Jerusalem artichokes, shallots, onion powder	May improve quality of intestinal microflora

Fructo-oligosaccharides

Saponins	Soya beans, soya foods, protein-containing foods	May lower LDL cholesterol; contains anti-cancer enzymes

Sulfides/Thiols

Diallyl sulfide	Onion, garlic, olives, leeks, spring onions, cruciferous vegetables	Lower LDL cholesterol, maintain healthy immune system
Allyl methyl trisulfide		
Dithoilthiones		

Source: International Food Information Council

Living a Vegetarian Lifestyle

Like millions of others, you may have chosen to lead a vegetarian lifestyle. Most people who have made such food choices will find that a vegetarian lifestyle fits perfectly with the Slim•Fast Makeover.* Vegetarian diets tend to be rich in fibre, complex carbohydrates and many vitamins and minerals, including the antioxidants vitamin C and beta-carotene. Although you may eat less protein than a non-vegetarian, chances are you're getting enough to meet the RDA for protein. Some vegetarians may be at risk for deficiencies in iron, calcium, copper, zinc, manganese, or vitamin B12. Fortunately, the Slim•Fast products are all fortified with these vitamins and minerals as well as protein. Using two Slim•Fast meal replacements a day and a carefully planned sensible meal should ensure that you have adequate amounts of the nutrients you need. The following foods are good sources for bolstering your intake of nutrients usually obtained from animal proteins:

- Protein: lentils, tofu, nuts, seeds, tempeh, peas
- Iron: dried beans, spinach, chard, molasses, bulgur, dried fruit
- Calcium: broccoli, kale, turnip greens, fortified soya milk or fruit juices, fortified tofu

* Slim•Fast products contain milk protein, so vegan dieters should take note.

Now that you've got the nutritional basics under your belt, you're ready to move on to designing your own personal makeover. It's time to transform your body and mind to get the life you've always wanted. This next chapter will give you the road map, but ultimately you're the one behind the wheel. Bon voyage!

6

designing your
own personal makeover

It's time to ask yourself: am I ready to take charge of my life? Am I ready to become the master of my weight, my body and my future?

Whether or not you're aware of it, you've already taken the reins. The 14-Day Plan showed you how it's done; you've learned the basics of nutrition and why the plan works. Now it's time to do it yourself.

When you give yourself the Slim•Fast Makeover, you'll be doing just that. *You* will choose the foods you eat, the exercises you do and the ways you manage stress. You will map out a personal makeover that fits into your own unique lifestyle.

Of course, you have to follow a basic framework. (You can't expect to lose weight if you exercise only five minutes a day or eat a huge slice of cheesecake for dessert every night!) The next two chapters give you the rules of the Slim•Fast Makeover, and show you how to get started.

Although there are rules to follow, you'll have a lot of flexibility in the options you choose – from what you eat to how you exercise to what kinds of relaxation techniques are best for you. Having the freedom to personalize your own makeover will make it easier to stay on the plan for good. It's a plan you'll be happy to live with; you won't even *want* to drop it once you reach your goal.

If you've ever seen a cosmetic makeover on a TV chat show, you must have wondered what happened after the cameras were turned off and the subject went home to try to re-create her new look. After all, she would no longer have the benefit of professionals to maintain that new look. The trouble with many beauty makeovers is that stylists don't teach the subject the skills she needs to transform herself day after day. And they usually don't think to do a makeover that can be easily replicated under a tight schedule and budget.

Allowing you to design a plan that fits into your life and giving you the tools to follow through with it – these are exactly the goals of the Slim•Fast Makeover. Rather than seeing the results of your makeover in the blink of an eye – and watching them fade just as fast – you'll see a steady transformation. You'll gradually take off weight and see a sculpted body begin to emerge. You'll notice that you have a little more energy each day, and find that you actually start to *crave* physical activity. You'll begin to have more confidence in yourself until you feel like you can accomplish anything.

How to Design Your Personal Makeover

You'll be designing three distinct plans that should fit easily into your daily lifestyle: an eating plan, an exercise plan and a relaxation plan. In this chapter, you'll be designing your eating plan. In the next chapter, you'll be designing a plan for exercise and relaxation, which work hand in hand to reduce stress, boost energy and help you feel great about your body and your life. The key to making the Slim•Fast Makeover work for you is choosing the recipes and lifestyle activities you enjoy most; that's what the Slim•Fast Makeover is all about – finding your own way.

Once you've begun creating your personal plan, you'll need to keep track of your progress. The best way to do this is to keep a personal makeover diary. Each day you should write down every-thing you've eaten, along with your estimated total calorie count. You should also make note of the exercise you did (and your esti-mated calorie burn) and the relaxation techniques you used. You should also record your daily weight, and make general notes – on recipes you liked, whether a particular workout felt great or seemed too strenuous, and so on. *Keeping a daily workout diary is a vital part of this plan.* It allows you to see what works and what doesn't. It also lets you know whether you've suffered a lapse here or there by not getting enough exercise or by over indulging.

Creating Your Personal Eating Plan

After following the 14-Day Plan, you're probably in one of two places: either you've lost weight and want to lose some more, or you've lost weight and want to maintain the loss. Most likely, you fall into the first category – which means you'll be creating a weight-loss eating plan. At some point (whether you're there now or later), you'll reach your goal weight – at which point you can design a weight-maintenance plan to help keep it off for life.

Weight-Loss Eating Plan

To lose weight, you'll be on a 1,400- to 1,500-calorie-a-day plan that gives you two Slim•Fast shakes or four meal replacement bars instead of two regular meals, just as you had on the 14-Day Plan. Your goal should be to lose ½–1 kilogram (1–2 pounds) per week. (Some dieters may need to eat slightly more or less than what is on the plan to achieve this slow but steady weight loss; see below for details.)

And here's where the variety kicks in: for your third meal, you can choose from among the dozens of recipes in this chapter. For instance, if you decide to have a shake for breakfast and another for lunch, you can choose a recipe that is suitable as an evening meal. If the next day you decide to have a shake for breakfast and dinner, you can whip up a quick and delicious recipe for lunch. To control hunger between meals, you should also have two or three daily snacks between meals. Choose a Slim•Fast snack bar, or a snack from the list on the following pages.

REMEMBER, FOR WEIGHT LOSS IT'S:

Shake • Shake • Meal

BREAKFAST: Slim•Fast Shake or 2 Meal Replacement Bars
SNACK: 1 piece of fruit, 115g/4oz raw vegetables, or a 60–90 calorie snack
LUNCH: Slim•Fast Shake or 2 Meal Replacement Bars
SNACK: 1 piece of fruit, 115g/4oz raw vegetables, or a 60–90 calorie snack
SNACK: Slim•Fast Snack Bar or a 100–150 calorie snack
DINNER: Large tossed salad; 170g/6oz of protein (meat, chicken, fish, or soya/vegetable protein); 3 servings of cooked vegetables; 1 serving starch (½ baked potato, 1 small corn on the cob, or 85g/3oz rice/pasta); 1 piece of fruit for dessert
BEVERAGES: Drink 8 glasses of water each day, and an extra glass for every caffeinated beverage you also consume

If you are small-framed or have been advised by your doctor to consume fewer calories per day, you can adjust the plan from 1,400 calories a day to 1,200. Reduce the size of your main protein source at dinner to 115g/4oz of lean meat, fish, poultry, or vegetable protein and have two snacks daily instead of three.

Note: You should be losing about ½–1 kilogram (1–2 pounds) per week, the healthiest way to lose weight. If you are losing more than that, you should eat more to slow the rate of weight loss. Start by adding one extra snack a day and adding an extra serving of starch with your meal. Continue to increase by this amount until your weight loss slows to the recommended amount.

Weight-Maintenance Eating Plan

To maintain your weight after you've reached your goal, you should be consuming about 300–500 calories more than you were consuming on the weight-loss plan. On the flip side, you should be consuming about 300–500 calories *less* than you were eating before you lost the weight. The easiest way to do this is to replace one Slim•Fast shake or two meal replacement bars with a second sensible meal. You'll continue to have one shake or two meal replacement bars each day for breakfast, lunch, or dinner, and then eat sensibly the rest of the day. You should also continue to have two or three daily snacks between meals.

FOR WEIGHT MAINTENANCE, IT'S:

Meal • Shake • Meal

BREAKFAST: 45g/1½oz high-fibre cereal, 250ml/8fl oz skimmed milk, 1 piece fruit *or* 1 Slim•Fast Shake or 2 Meal Replacement Bars

SNACK: 1 piece of fruit, 115g/4oz raw vegetables, or a 60–90 calorie snack

LUNCH: 1 sandwich (55g/2oz cold meat or cheese, 3 tomato slices, 2 lettuce leaves, 70g/2½oz grated carrot, 2 slices bread); 225g/8oz artificially sweetened virtually fat-free yogurt or 1 piece of fruit or 1 Slim•Fast Shake or 2 Meal Replacement Bars

SNACK: 1 piece of fruit, 115g/4oz raw vegetables, or a 60–90 calorie snack

SNACK: 1 Slim•Fast Snack Bar or a 100–150 calorie snack

DINNER: Vegetable soup or side salad; 170g/6oz of protein (meat, chicken, fish, or soya/vegetable protein); 3 servings of steamed or grilled vegetables; 1 serving of starch (potato, rice, pasta, etc.); 1 piece of fruit for dessert

BEVERAGES: Drink 8 glasses of water each day, and one extra glass for every caffeinated beverage you also consume

Slim•Fast Shakes and Bars – The Cornerstone of the Plan

Here's a list of Slim•Fast products you can use to replace meals or snacks. The shakes and meal replacement bars can be used in place of a breakfast, lunch, or dinner; the snack bars help fill in between meals.

Slim•Fast Powders

Chocolate Royale	Banana Deluxe	French Vanilla
Hot Chocolate	Strawberry Supreme	

Slim•Fast Ready to Drink Shakes

Coffee Delight	Strawberry Supreme	Chocolate Royale
Banana Deluxe	French Vanilla	

Slim•Fast Meal Replacement Bars

Chocolate Sensation   Toffee Delight

Slim•Fast Snack Bars

Chocolate Chip   Chocolate Muesli

Sensible Snacks

Making smart snack choices will give you energy during the day,
help satisfy your appetite and help you reach your weight-loss goal.
Snacking on fresh fruits and vegetables will give you the most nutrition in the fewest amount of calories. Still, sometimes you may want
to snack on something a little more substantial. Here are some
snacks that won't sabotage your weight-loss efforts. Enjoy two
snacks from the 60- to 90-calorie category and one from the 100- to
150-calorie category each day.

60 to 90 Calories

1 piece fresh fruit
125ml/4fl oz fruit juice
115g/4 oz blueberries
15g/½ oz 99% fat-free pretzels
55g/2oz air-popped popcorn
3 lightly salted crispy crackers

3 Marie biscuits
30g/1oz dried apricots
20g packet apple chips
3 sesame seed breadsticks
150g/5½ oz fruit cocktail in
    fruit juice

100 to 150 Calories

1 Slim•Fast Snack Bar

200g tub virtually fat-free yogurt

4 slices light rye crispbread

½ bagel with 1 tablespoon
   all-fruit spread

295g can low-fat soup

85g/3oz frozen low fat yogurt

150g pot low-fat creamed rice

2 oatcakes with 2 teaspoons
   low-fat cottage cheese

1 medium banana

45g/1½ oz mozzarella cheese

85g/3oz fruit sorbet

1 Geobar (cereal bar)

Your Weekly Shopping List

How many times have you had to forgo trying a new recipe because you were missing a few essential ingredients? You'll see that it pays to plan ahead and outline a weekly menu for yourself. Look over the recipes on the following pages and think about what you want to prepare for the coming week. Check your kitchen for what you already have, then compose a shopping list with all the ingredients you'll need to get on your next trip to the supermarket.

Guide to Supermarket Shopping

Here's one thing you should know: your supermarket shopping habits can make or break your weight-loss goals. The simple lessons you've always heard still hold: never shop when you're hungry; shop with a food list; and don't buy your favourite binge foods 'for the family', because you'll end up eating them, too. As you're composing your shopping list, move mentally through the aisles and think about what's available in every section. Divide your list into sections and consider the pros and cons of the possibilities that await you.

Fresh Produce Gazing upon row after row of brilliantly-coloured fruits and vegetables, give in to the temptation to try an unusual squash or a new variety of salad leaf. This is the only area of the supermarket where it pays to be decadent. Getting a colourful array of fruits and vegetables will give you a greater variety of phytochemicals. And don't hurry through this section. Allow yourself time to inspect the produce, seeing what looks good. Fresh vegetables won't break your budget (if you buy those that are in season) and are ideal for boosting your health and your weight-loss efforts.

Canned and Packaged Goods Spend the least amount of time in these aisles, where the processed foods beckon. You'll find eye-catching packaging and 'special offers' but don't be tempted into buying what you don't need. Steer clear of processed meals as much as possible as they are often loaded with sodium, fat and calories. In general, buy things as minimally processed as possible: low-sodium, whole-grain, high-fibre items.

Meats, Fish and Poultry You can save money if you buy these pricier items in bulk or when they're on special offer. Set aside what you need over the next few days and freeze the rest. Choose meats with the smallest amount of visible fat. Boneless roasts, chops and skinless poultry may be more expensive, but are less wasteful. To get the freshest fish, ask if the fish was delivered that day or (at the latest) the day before. Don't rule out frozen cuts. If there's no sign of dryness (or ice crystals, which can indicate thawing), they're often fresher and cheaper than what's on the fish counter.

The Deli Counter and Packaged Meats You'll need to navigate this area very carefully. Use restraint, and don't buy anything swimming in mayonnaise or oil. Don't be fooled into thinking that pasta salads, tuna salad and oily vegetables are 'salads' in the healthy sense of the word. They are havens for hidden fat and calories. Ditto for the savoury pastries, stuffed peppers and other prepared dishes that may tempt you with their ease and convenience. (Save the calories for when you go out for a meal.)

Frozen Foods It's easy to be seduced by the ice-cream, cakes and desserts in these aisles. Bypass them for healthier options. Unsweetened frozen fruit can make a great dessert, or can be puréed into a quick sauce. Fruit sorbets are also a good low-calorie snack options, as are low-fat ice-cream and frozen yogurt – always remember, however, the low-fat label is not a licence to overeat. If you can steer clear of these areas and head straight for the frozen vegetables, so much the better. *Frozen vegetables* provide an easy and convenient way to getting your vegetable quota for the day. Variety packs of three or more vegetables like broccoli, corn, carrots and green beans are particularly good if you run out of fresh produce. *Frozen ready-made dinners* can also be useful if you don't have time to prepare your own. Look for low-fat, vegetable-heavy makes like Healthy Choice or Lean Cuisine. On the Slim•Fast Plan, you should be eating about around 600 calories for dinner, so you may need to eat two of these to get a full meal.

Dairy This is often a tricky area, as many people adore dairy produce. Thankfully there are far more low-fat options available than there were just a few years ago and as always you can have that treat – just do it in moderation. *Full-flavoured cheeses such as Parmesan and Roquefort* are useful as you only need a little bit to get the desired flavour. For your everyday needs, however, go for *low-fat options* in the dairy section – skimmed milk, diet margarine, reduced-fat cheeses. Very low fat yogurt and low-fat cottage cheese are also readily available – go for the plain, unflavoured versions to get the most versatility. You can cut your own fresh fruit into cottage cheese, and use fresh herbs to make a tasty yogurt dip for your vegetables.

Bakery The bakery aisle offers too many goodies, and the smells of freshly baked goods can be very enticing. Still, there are healthy items here – if you steer clear of the cakes and cookies. Freshly-baked bread, in particular, is often as enticing as the cakes, but be careful with your choice. Hi-fibre is best, so go for the wholemeal option and not the crusty white. It is difficult to tell just how high-fibre a bread is – whole-grain and wholemeal don't necessarily mean high-fibre, so ask. The task is simpler when you're buying packaged bread – look for one where each slice contains 3 grams or more of fibre. Also, look for brands that are reduced-calorie, so you can have two slices of bread for the same number of calories as one.

A note on packaged soups and salad dressings: many brands of commercially prepared low-fat soups and salad dressings are available on store shelves. When shopping for these items, look carefully at the Nutritional Information panel. For *low-fat soups,* select those with 3 grams or less of fat per serving, with 1 gram or less saturated fat. Also, look at sodium content, which is often very high in canned soups. Look out for 'healthy' low-fat varieties with 475 mg or less of sodium per serving.

Commercial salad dressings are available as reduced-fat, lite, low-calorie, and fat-free. Look for those with 0 grams of saturated fat per serving (serving size is 2 tablespoons). Again, sodium content may often be very high; however, there are brands available with lower sodium content that are fat-free *and* tasty.

Discovering the Kitchen

A great gift this Slim•Fast life has given me is ... the art of cooking! I've always *wanted* to cook well, and I've often fooled myself into thinking I knew what I was doing – at least until an Italian painter friend of mine teased me once: 'Lauren, you *act* cooking.'

Well, you can only get away with acting for so long (at least until you have to throw a dinner party). So now, after having a Slim•Fast shake for breakfast and lunch, by dinner I'm ready to *eat*. And I'm not taking any chances on messing anything up. For the first time in my life, I'm following recipes closely – and creating some of my own! No more half-baked shortcuts, no more talking on the phone or wandering off to read a book midstream. Now I stick to the business at hand – and the results are delicious.

Stocking the Kitchen

Now that I've become so much more interested in cooking, here's a quick sketch of all the wonderful things I keep on hand in my kitchen *at all times* – a host of great foodstuffs that makes it easy to eat healthy every day.

Filter jug full of water

Raw (unprocessed) apple and cranberry juice

Red grapefruit

The berries – blue, black, rasp

Lemons and limes

Cucumbers

Broccoli

Tons of garlic

Firm tofu

Pasta in all varieties (I buy the fresh varieties)

Low-sodium chicken stock

Rice – brown and basmati

Bulgur wheat

Polenta

Organic tomatoes and plum
    tomatoes
Yellow and spaghetti squash
Carrots
Celery
Radishes
Bean sprouts
Sweet Bermuda onions
Red onions
Chillies – habaneros and
    jalapeños
Shiitake mushrooms
Lettuce (any kind)
Fresh spinach
Endive
Italian parsley
Coriander
Spring onions
Shallots
Fresh root ginger
Fresh horseradish

Dried beans – split pea, green
    and yellow, cannellini, black
    and black-eyed, flageolets;
    kidneys
Wild white sage honey
Every spice I can get my hands
    on – whole or powdered.
    Buy in small quantities and
    bottle them yourself; don't
    forget to replace them if
    they get too old (after a year
    or so)
Low-fat flour or corn tortillas
Black olive paste
Sweet pepper paste
Good Parmesan cheese (whole,
    not pre-grated)
Extra-virgin olive oil
White peach and mint tea
Six-pack of Slim•Fast in the
    fridge

The Recipes

The recipes are divided into a series of menus, each one categorized according to the central ingredient of the main course. Each main course recipe is followed by recipes or suggestions for suitable accompaniments and fruit to finish. Where the main recipe is accompanied by a packaged item (such as crackers or yogurt), look for a product with a very similar nutritional value to that listed.

Chicken and Turkey

Warm Chicken and Vegetable Salad

•

Mediterranean Chicken Pockets

•

Chicken and Tagliatelle Dijon

•

Honey-Grilled Chicken Breast

•

Turkey-Stuffed Pitta Breads

•

Turkey Fajitas

•

Turkey Breast Steaks with Cranberry Sauce

Menu

Warm Chicken and Vegetable Salad
Sautéed Portobello Mushrooms
Wholemeal crackers
Cantaloupe melon wedge

Warm Chicken and Vegetable Salad

SERVES 4   total preparation time: **60 minutes**

2 large floury potatoes, peeled and sliced 2.5cm/1 inch thick
450g/1lb fresh green beans, trimmed and cut into 5cm/2 inch
    pieces
Nonstick cooking spray
780g/1¾ lb boneless, skinless chicken breasts, cut into 5cm/2 inch
    pieces
2 large tomatoes, quartered
1 small red onion, diced
115g/4oz 90% fat-free mayonnaise-style dressing
1 tablespoon lemon juice
½ teaspoon thyme
½ teaspoon tarragon
¼ teaspoon salt
½ teaspoon pepper
1 head cos lettuce, leaves separated

1. Fill a large saucepan with enough water to cover potatoes and
    bring to the boil. Add potatoes to boiling water, reduce heat to
    medium and cook 15–20 minutes, until tender when pierced
    with a fork. Drain, cool and dice.

2. Meanwhile, fill a medium saucepan with 5cm/2 inches water and bring to the boil. Put cut green beans in steamer or colander, place in saucepan and steam 5 minutes, or until crisp-tender.

3. Spray a large nonstick frying pan with cooking spray and warm over medium heat. Add chicken and sauté 5–8 minutes, turning frequently, until thoroughly cooked and no longer pink inside.

4. In a large mixing bowl, combine cooked chicken, diced potatoes, steamed green beans, tomato quarters and diced onion. Add mayonnaise, lemon juice, thyme, tarragon, salt and pepper, and blend well.

5. Place lettuce leaves on serving plates. Top with warm chicken and vegetable mixture and serve with 4 wholemeal crackers per portion.

Sautéed Portobello Mushrooms

SERVES 4   total preparation time: **15 minutes**

Nonstick cooking spray
450g/1lb portobello or flat mushrooms, cut into 1cm/½ inch-thick
    slices
3 tablespoons Worcestershire sauce
½ teaspoon ground black pepper
15g/½ oz chopped parsley

Spray a large nonstick frying pan with cooking spray. Add mushrooms and Worcestershire sauce and sauté 5–7 minutes over medium heat, until mushrooms are soft. Add pepper and parsley and cook 2–3 minutes. Drain excess moisture, remove to a plate and serve.

nutritional information per serving

	Calories	Protein	Carbs	Fat	Fibre	Sodium	Cholesterol	Calcium
Warm Chicken Salad								
	505	55 g	36 g	16 g	6 g	491 mg	143 mg	98 mg
Sautéed Flat Mushrooms								
	42	4 g	6 g	2 g	2 g	132 mg	0 mg	23 mg
4 wholemeal crackers								
	35	0.5 g	5 g	1.5 g	1 g	50 mg	0 mg	4 mg
Cantaloupe wedge (⅛ melon)								
	24	1 g	6 g	0.5 g	0.5 g	6 mg	0 mg	8 mg
Meal Total								
	606	60.5 g	53 g	20 g (29%)*	9.5 g	679 mg	143 mg	133 mg

*Percentage of calories from fat

Mediterranean Chicken Pockets

SERVES 4   **total preparation time: 18 minutes**

Nonstick cooking spray

1 teaspoon rapeseed oil

680g/1½ lb boneless, skinless chicken breasts, cut into 1cm/½ inch
    pieces

285g/10oz frozen peas

2 medium tomatoes, chopped

55g/2oz feta cheese, crumbled

1 spring onion, chopped

170g/6oz very low fat natural yogurt

55g/2oz 90% fat-free mayonnaise-style dressing

1 tablespoon lemon juice

2 teaspoons chopped fresh dill

Four 45g/1½ oz pitta breads, sliced open

½ small head iceberg lettuce, separated into leaves

1. Spray a large nonstick frying pan with cooking spray, brush with
    oil and place over medium-high heat. Add chicken pieces and
    sauté, turning frequently, until cooked and no longer pink inside,
    5–6 minutes. Remove to a plate, cover and allow to cool in refrig-
    erator.

2. Meanwhile, bring 125ml/4fl oz water to the boil in a medium saucepan and add frozen peas. Bring to the boil, reduce heat, cover and simmer 4 minutes; do not overcook. Drain and set aside.

3. In a large bowl, combine chicken, cooked peas, tomatoes, feta cheese and spring onion. Fold in yogurt, mayonnaise dressing, lemon juice and dill, and toss well.

4. Line inside of pitta halves with lettuce and stuff with chicken mixture.

Quick Carrot Slaw

SERVES 4   total preparation time: **10–12 minutes**

4 large carrots, grated
1 small red onion, thinly sliced
60ml/2fl oz cider or apple juice
2 tablespoons reduced-fat mayonnaise
2 tablespoons cider vinegar
½ teaspoon granulated artificial sweetener
¼ teaspoon salt
¼ teaspoon ground pepper

Food-processor method: Combine all ingredients in food processor, and pulse 4 or 5 times until all ingredients are finely chopped and blended together. *Hand method:* After grating carrot and slicing onion, chop very finely. Place all ingredients in medium mixing bowl and stir until well blended. Transfer to a serving bowl, cover and chill before serving.

nutritional information per serving

	Calories	Protein	Carbs	Fat	Fibre	Sodium	Cholesterol	Calcium
Mediterranean Chicken Pockets								
	528	49 g	46 g	18 g	6 g	794 mg	116 mg	206 mg
Quick Carrot Slaw								
	85	1.5 g	18 g	2 g	4 g	223 mg	2 mg	38 mg
Grapes (about 15)								
	53	0.5 g	13 g	0.5 g	1 g	2 mg	0 mg	8 mg
Meal Total								
	666	51 g	77 g	20.5 g (27%)	11 g	1,019 mg	118 mg	252 mg

Leslie Schultz

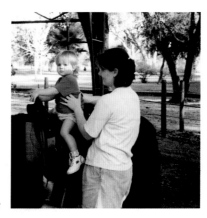

Before

After

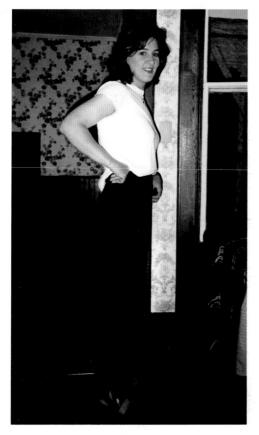

Leslie Schultz is a registered nurse who recently lost over 20 pounds (9 kilos) on Slimfast. 'The diet worked so well for me that there are at least six other nurses on my unit who are also on it now. All the nurses thanked me for turning them on to Slimfast and for encouraging them.'

Lisa
Custard

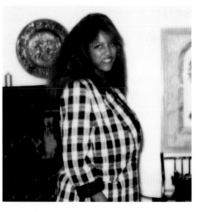

Before

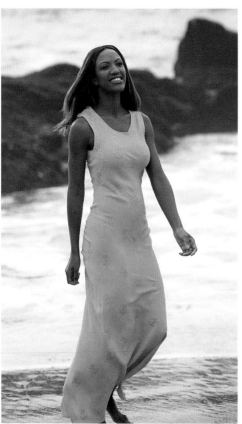

After

Lisa Custard was thrilled by her own Slimfast success story – which led to her being featured on a television commercial. 'A yummy, healthy shake that fills you up. Who could ask for anything more? I used to be 35 pounds (16 kilos) overweight, but by using Slimfast I've lost the weight and kept it off for over two years. My attitude has changed as well; I never used to smile, but now I smile so much the only thing I have to worry about is getting laugh lines around my mouth.'

Katie
Taggart

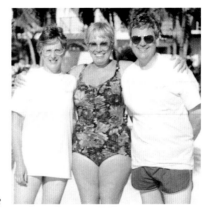

Before

After

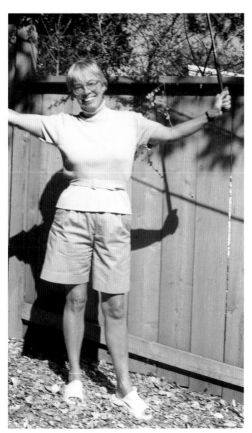

Katie Taggart, a
sixty-year-old
saleswoman, reached
her weight-loss goal
in twelve weeks; she
now weighs 35
pounds (16 kilos)
less. 'I can get into
clothes from seven
years ago,' she says.
'I only wonder why
I didn't start the
programme
much earlier.'

Andy
Fischer

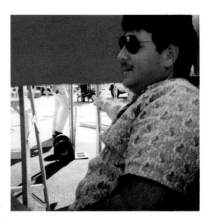

Before

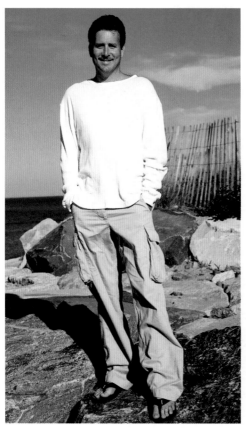

After

Andy Fischer, a TV cameraman and diving aficionado, lost 43 pounds (19 kilos) on the Slimfast Plan – which he discovered while he was shooting Slimfast commercials featuring other successful dieters. 'When I put on a wetsuit,' he remembers, it was a bad situation – I was fat.' Today his life is different. 'I'm ecstatic about what I've done for myself. I can't tell you how good I feel – I feel young and rejuvenated. Right now I have the energy to do anything.'

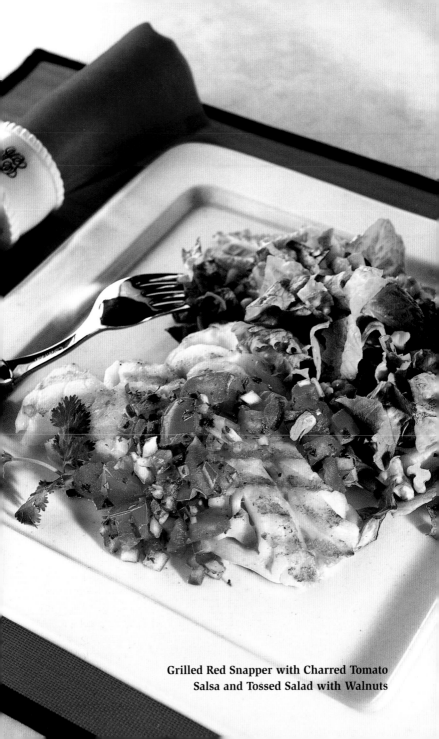

Grilled Red Snapper with Charred Tomato
Salsa and Tossed Salad with Walnuts

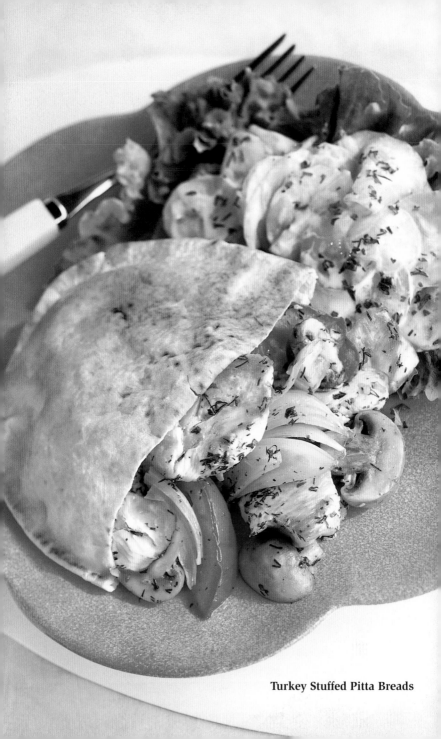

Turkey Stuffed Pitta Breads

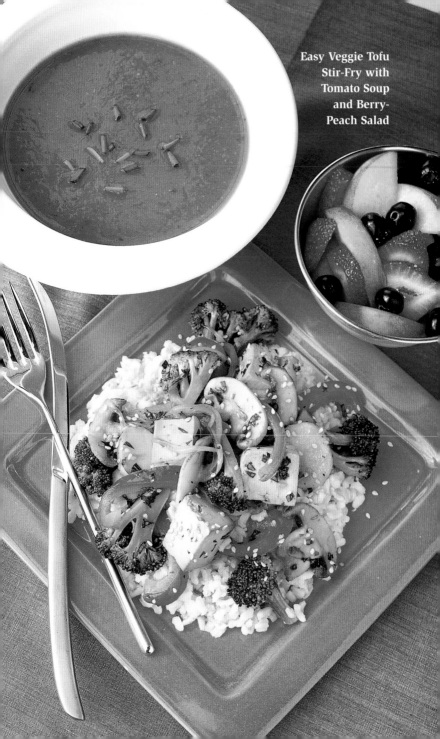

Easy Veggie Tofu Stir-Fry with Tomato Soup and Berry-Peach Salad

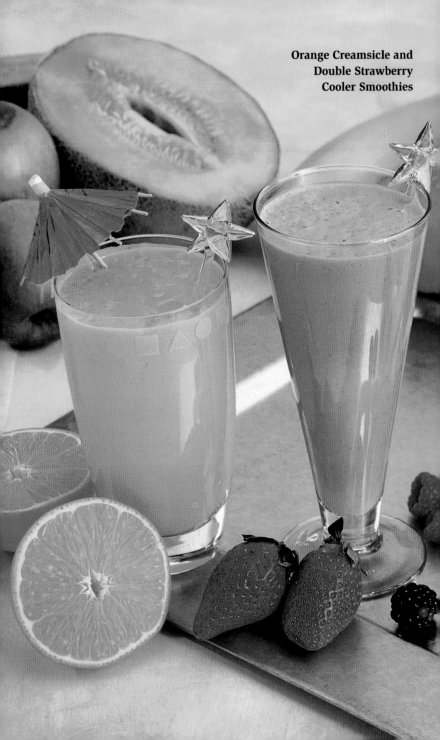

Orange Creamsicle and Double Strawberry Cooler Smoothies

Menu

Chicken and Tagliatelle Dijon
Rosemary-Steamed Broccoli and Carrots
Tossed Salad with Tomatoes
Medium fresh orange

Chicken and Tagliatelle Dijon

SERVES 4 **total preparation time: 20–25 minutes**

225g/8oz very low fat natural yogurt
1½ tablespoons Dijon mustard
½ teaspoon dried thyme
Four 200g/7oz boneless, skinless chicken breasts, cut into bite-size
   pieces
Nonstick cooking spray
225g/8oz button mushrooms, thinly sliced
2 tablespoons water
170g/6oz tagliatelle
½ lemon, sliced very thin
½ teaspoon freshly ground black pepper

1. In a small bowl, stir together yogurt, mustard and thyme.
2. Spray a large nonstick frying pan with cooking spray. Place on
   medium heat and add chicken. Sauté, stirring frequently, 5–6
   minutes, or until chicken is cooked through and no longer pink.
   Remove chicken from pan to a plate, cover and keep warm. Add
   mushrooms and 2 tablespoons water to the pan, cover and cook
   over medium heat until soft, about 2 minutes. Add yogurt mixture to mushrooms and heat, but do *not* boil. Return chicken to
   pan and gently mix with mushroom and yogurt sauce.

3. Meanwhile, bring 1.5 litres/2½ pints of water to boil in a large pot. Add tagliatelle and cook, stirring frequently, until al dente, 6–7 minutes or according to package directions. Remove from heat, drain, set aside and keep warm.

4. Place warm tagliatelle on a serving plate and top with chicken and sauce. Garnish with lemon slices and sprinkle with freshly ground pepper.

Tossed Salad with Tomatoes

SERVES 4   total preparation time: **10–12 minutes**

½ head cos lettuce, torn into bite-size pieces
½ head iceberg lettuce, torn into bite-size pieces
4 medium tomatoes, cut into small wedges
125ml/4fl oz fat-free salad dressing

Place lettuce in a large salad bowl and toss with tomato wedges. Dress immediately before serving.

Rosemary-Steamed Broccoli and Carrots

SERVES 4   total preparation time: **12 minutes**

1 tablespoon chopped fresh rosemary or 1 teaspoon dried
900g/2lb broccoli, cut into bite-size florets
450g/1lb carrots, sliced into 5mm/¼ inch pieces

Fill a large saucepan with 5cm/2 inches water and bring to the boil. Add chopped rosemary to water and reduce heat to simmer. Place broccoli and carrots in a steamer over water and steam 5 minutes, or until crisp-tender.

nutritional information per serving

	Calories	Protein	Carbs	Fat	Fibre	Sodium	Cholesterol	Calcium
Chicken and Tagliatelle Dijon								
	450	57 g	40 g	5.5 g	2 g	331 mg	154 mg	128 mg
Rosemary- Steamed Broccoli and Carrots								
	89	5 g	19 g	1 g	8 g	77 mg	0 mg	103 mg
Tossed Salad with Tomatoes								
	70	3 g	15 g	1 g	4 g	38 mg	0 mg	52 mg
Medium fresh orange								
	62	1 g	15 g	0 g	3 g	0 mg	0 mg	52 mg
Meal Total								
	671	66 g	89 g	7.5 g (10%)	17 g	446 mg	154 mg	335 mg

Honey-Grilled Chicken Breast
Tossed Salad
Sliced apple with cinnamon
Baked Sweet Potato
Oregano-Scented Summer Squash
Steamed Spinach
Parsley Carrot Coins

Honey-Grilled Chicken Breast

SERVES 4   **total preparation time: 45 minutes**

1 tablespoon orange juice

2 teaspoons lemon juice

2 teaspoons honey

2 teaspoons light (reduced-sodium) soy sauce

1 teaspoon grated fresh root ginger

1 clove garlic, crushed

Four 200g/7oz boneless, skinless chicken breasts

1. Combine all ingredients except chicken in large shallow dish and whisk until blended. Add chicken breasts, turn several times to coat, cover with clingfilm and place in refrigerator. Marinate 15 minutes or up to 1 hour.
2. Preheat the grill. Place chicken in grill pan and grill 4–5 minutes per side, or until cooked through and juices run clear. They are also delicious cooked on a barbecue.
3. Remove to a plate and allow to stand 5 minutes before serving.

Tossed Salad

SERVES 4   total preparation time: **10 minutes**

1 small head cos lettuce, torn into bite-size pieces
1 small head red-leaf lettuce, torn into bite-size pieces
     24 cherry tomatoes, halved
1 small red onion, thinly sliced
12 button mushrooms, thinly sliced
125ml/4fl oz fat-free salad dressing

Toss all ingredients, except dressing, in a large salad bowl. Dress immediately before serving.

Baked Sweet Potato

SERVES 4   total preparation time: **5–8 or 50–60 minutes, depending on method**

2 medium sweet potatoes, with skin (see Note),
     scrubbed well, ends trimmed

Oven method: Preheat oven to 200°C/400°F/Gas mark 6. Prick potatoes a few times with a fork. Place on baking sheet and bake 50–60 minutes, or until soft when pierced by a fork. *Microwave method:* Prick potatoes twice with a fork. Place side by side in centre of microwave oven. Cook on high 5–8 minutes, or until soft when pierced with a fork.

Note: The skin of sweet potatoes contains many nutrients and fibre and should be left on and eaten whenever possible.

Oregano-Scented Summer Squash

SERVES 4   total preparation time: **10 minutes**

1 teaspoon dried or 1 tablespoon fresh chopped oregano
450g/1lb yellow summer squash, trimmed and cut into 1cm/½ inch
  slices

Fill a large saucepan with 5cm/2 inches water and bring to the
boil. Add oregano. Place summer squash in steamer or colander
and place in saucepan. Steam 5 minutes, or until crisp-tender.

Steamed Spinach

SERVES 4   total preparation time: **10 minutes**

900g/2lb fresh spinach, tough ends removed, washed thoroughly

Fill a large saucepan with 5cm/2 inches water and bring to the
boil. Place spinach in steamer or colander and place in saucepan.
Steam spinach 5 minutes, or until wilted but still bright green.

Parsley Carrot Coins

SERVES 4   **total preparation time: 15 minutes**

450g/1lb carrots, cut into 5mm/¼ inch slices
2 tablespoons chopped fresh parsley

Fill a large saucepan with 5cm/2 inches water and bring to the
boil. Place carrots in steamer or colander and place in saucepan.
Steam 8–10 minutes, or until crisp-tender. Toss with parsley and
serve.

nutritional information per serving

	Calories	Protein	Carbs	Fat	Fibre	Sodium	Cholesterol	Calcium
Honey-Grilled Chicken Breast								
	298	43 g	4 g	11 g	0 g	202 mg	120 mg	23 mg
Tossed Salad								
	88	5 g	18 g	1 g	5 g	35 mg	0 mg	73 mg
Baked Sweet Potato								
	59	1 g	14 g	0 g	2 g	6 mg	0 mg	16 mg
Oregano-Scented Summer Squash								
	23	1 g	5 g	0 g	2 g	2 mg	0 mg	27 mg
Steamed Spinach								
	36	5 g	6 g	0.5 g	4 g	129 mg	0 mg	162 mg
Parsley Carrot Coins								
	49	1 g	12 g	0	3 g	41 mg	0 mg	33 mg
Sliced Apple (1 medium)								
	81	0 g	21 g	0.5 g	4 g	0 mg	0 mg	10 mg
Meal Total								
	634	56 g	89 g	13 g (18%)	20 g	415 mg	120 mg	344 mg

Turkey-Stuffed Pitta Breads
Cucumber-Yogurt Salad
Nectarine

Turkey-Stuffed Pitta Breads

SERVES 4   **total preparation time: 1 hour**

1 tablespoon finely chopped fresh dill

1 teaspoon dried oregano

4 cloves garlic, crushed

¼ teaspoon ground black pepper

780g/1¾ lb turkey breast meat, cut into 5cm/2 inch cubes

3 large onions, cut into wedges

3 large tomatoes, cut into wedges

12 large button mushrooms, halved

Four 17cm/6½-inch pitta breads

1. Combine dill, oregano, garlic and pepper in a small mixing bowl. Place turkey pieces in a shallow dish, sprinkle with half the spice mixture and toss to coat. Cover and marinate 15 minutes or up to 1 hour in the refrigerator.

2. Preheat oven to 220°C/425°F/Gas mark 7.

3. In a medium mixing bowl, toss the remaining half of the spice mix with the onions, tomatoes and mushrooms.

4. Prepare foil packets: using two large sheets of aluminium foil, place half the marinated turkey in the centre of each and surround with vegetables. Bring up the sides of the foil and double fold. Then double fold the ends to form a packet, leaving 5cm/ 2 inches on each end for heat circulation.

5. Place on a baking sheet and cook in the oven for 25 minutes.
6. Split pitta breads in half and stuff with the turkey and vegetables.

Cucumber-Yogurt Salad

SERVES 4   total preparation time: **30–60 minutes**

4 medium cucumbers, peeled and thinly sliced
1 teaspoon salt
450g/16oz very low fat natural yogurt
1 head red- or green-leaf lettuce, shredded

1. Place sliced cucumbers in a large mixing bowl and add salt. Mix and allow to stand 5 minutes.
2. Pat cucumbers dry using kitchen paper. Add yogurt and toss well to coat. Cover and refrigerate 15 minutes or up to 45 minutes.
3. Arrange lettuce leaves on individual plates and top with cucumber mixture.

nutritional information per serving

	Calories	Protein	Carbs	Fat	Fibre	Sodium	Cholesterol	Calcium
Turkey-Stuffed Pitta Breads								
	471	60 g	50 g	3 g	5 g	426 mg	141 mg	122 mg
Cucumber- Yogurt Salad								
	94	8 g	19 g	0.5 g	3 g	657 mg	3 mg	205 mg
Nectarine (1 medium)								
	66	1 g	16 g	1 g	2 g	0 mg	0 mg	7 mg
Meal Total								
	631	69 g	85 g	4.5 (13%)	10 g	1,083 mg	144 mg	334 mg

Turkey Fajitas
Mixed Green Salad (page 151)
Sliced papaya

Turkey Fajitas

SERVES 4   total preparation time: **20 minutes**

Nonstick cooking spray
780g/1¾ lb stir-fry turkey meat
3 teaspoons olive oil
4 cloves garlic, crushed
2 medium yellow onions, thinly sliced
1 medium red pepper, cored and sliced into strips
1 medium green pepper, cored and sliced into strips
½ teaspoon cumin
¼ teaspoon coriander
1 teaspoon oregano
1 teaspoon paprika
¼ teaspoon cayenne pepper
¾ teaspoon chilli powder
4 tablespoons very low fat natural yogurt
4 medium low-fat flour or corn tortillas (see Note)
55g/2oz salsa
30g/1oz 95% fat-free Cheddar-style cheese, grated

1. Spray a large nonstick frying pan with cooking spray. Place over medium heat, add turkey meat and sauté 5–8 minutes, turning frequently, until thoroughly cooked and no longer pink inside.

2. Remove turkey from pan and set aside, covered. Add olive oil, garlic and onions to pan. Sauté over medium heat until garlic is golden and onions translucent, 3–5 minutes.
3. Add red and green pepper strips, cumin, coriander, oregano, paprika, cayenne and chilli powder. Continue to cook, adding a little water if necessary, until peppers soften a little, 5–6 minutes.
4. Return cooked turkey strips to vegetable mixture and gently mix.
5. Spread yogurt on top of warm tortillas. Divide fajita mixture among the 4 tortillas and top each with 1 tablespoon salsa and a little cheese. Roll and serve warm.

Note: to warm tortillas in the microwave, place flat in microwave and heat on medium for 45–50 seconds until hot; do not over-heat. Oven method: wrap tortillas in aluminium foil and warm in a 130°C/250°F/Gas mark ½ oven for 10 minutes.

nutritional information per serving

	Calories	Protein	Carbs	Fat	Fibre	Sodium	Cholesterol	Calcium
Turkey Fajitas								
	591	53 g	42 g	22 g	5 g	577 mg	130 mg	221 mg
Mixed Green Salad								
	115	6 g	24 g	1 g	7 g	44 mg	0 mg	131 mg
Sliced papaya (½)								
	59	1 g	15 g	0 g	3 g	5 mg	0 mg	36 mg
Meal Total								
	765	60 g	81 g	23 g (27%)	15 g	626 mg	130 mg	388 mg

Turkey Breasts with Cranberry Sauce
Wild Rice
Green Beans
Mashed Butternut Squash with Brown Sugar
Mixed Garden Salad (page 151)
Cantaloupe melon wedge

Turkey Breasts with Cranberry Sauce

SERVES 4   total preparation time: **18 minutes**

800g/1¾ lb turkey breasts
½ teaspoon ground nutmeg
125ml/4fl oz fat-free chicken stock
1 tablespoon cornflour
150g/5oz whole cranberry sauce

1. Preheat grill.
2. Sprinkle the steaks lightly with nutmeg.
3. Place turkey breast steaks on grill pan 10–15cm/4–5 inches from heat and cook 3–4 minutes. Turn and cook 3–4 minutes more, until no longer pink.
4. Meanwhile, combine chicken stock and cornflour in a small saucepan. Simmer over medium heat, stirring frequently, until bubbly and thickened. Add cranberry sauce and cook, stirring constantly, 2 minutes.
5. Place grilled turkey breasts on serving plates, top with cranberry sauce and serve.

Wild Rice

SERVES 4   total preparation time: **1 hour**

100g/3½oz uncooked wild rice, rinsed

In a heavy saucepan, bring 1 litre/35fl oz of water to the boil. Add rice, reduce heat to very low, cover tightly and simmer gently for 30 minutes. Remove from heat and leave to stand 25–30 minutes, until rice reaches desired texture. Drain completely and serve warm.

Green Beans

SERVES 4   total preparation time: **15 minutes**

450g/1lb fresh green beans, cut into 5cm/2 inch pieces

Fill a medium saucepan with 5cm/2 inches water and bring to the boil. Place cut green beans in steamer or colander and place in saucepan. Steam 5 minutes, or until crisp-tender.

Mashed Butternut Squash with Brown Sugar

SERVES 4   total preparation time: **40–55 minutes**

2 medium butternut squash (about 450g/1lb), cut in half, with seeds
    and stringy parts removed
1 tablespoon brown sugar
⅛ teaspoon ground nutmeg
⅛ teaspoon ground cinnamon
¼ teaspoon grated orange peel (orange part only, with no white pith)

1. Preheat oven to 200°C/400°F/Gas mark 6.
2. In a shallow baking dish, place squash halves cut-side down. Cover with foil and bake 30–45 minutes, or until flesh is tender when pierced with a fork.
3. Remove from oven, peel and cut into cubes.
4. In a large bowl, combine cubed squash, brown sugar, nutmeg, cinnamon and orange peel. Mash together or, using an electric mixer, beat on medium speed until fluffy.

nutritional information per serving

	Calories	Protein	Carbs	Fat	Fibre	Sodium	Cholesterol	Calcium
Turkey Breasts with Cranberry Sauce								
	320	49 g	14 g	5 g	2 g	227 mg	126 mg	38 mg
Wild Rice								
	80	3 g	17 g	0 g	1 g	2 mg	0 mg	2 mg
Green Beans								
	34	2 g	8 g	0 g	3 g	3 mg	0 mg	45 mg
Mashed Butternut Squash with Brown Sugar								
	57	1 g	15 g	0 g	3 g	5 mg	0 mg	50 mg
Mixed Garden Salad								
	74	3 g	16 g	1 g	4 g	37 mg	0 mg	56 mg
Cantaloupe								
	24	1 g	6 g	0 g	0.5 g	6 mg	0 mg	8 mg
Meal Total								
	589	59 g	76 g	6 g (9%)	13.5 g	280 mg	126 mg	199 mg

Seafood

Curried Tuna Salad

•

Grilled Salmon with Penne Primavera

•

Seafood Strata

•

Grilled Red Snapper with Charred Tomato Salsa

•

Herb-Rubbed Grilled Tuna

•

Balsamic-Grilled Halibut Steak

•

Lemon-Pepper Sole

Curried Tuna Salad

SERVES 4   **total preparation time: 20 minutes**

Three 200g cans tuna in brine, drained and flaked
410g can unpeeled apricot halves, in juice, quartered
225g/8oz strawberries, hulled and thinly sliced
2 celery sticks, finely diced
55g/2oz 90% fat-free mayonnaise-style dressing
55g/2oz very low fat natural yogurt
½ teaspoon curry powder
2 tablespoons lemon juice
1 head red-leaf lettuce

1. In a large bowl, combine tuna with apricots, sliced strawberries
    and diced celery. Mix thoroughly.
2. In a small bowl, blend mayonnaise dressing with the yogurt,
    curry powder and lemon juice. Line 4 dinner plates with lettuce
    leaves, spoon tuna mixture onto plates and top with dressing.

nutritional information per serving

	Calories	Protein	Carbs	Fat	Fibre	Sodium	Cholesterol	Calcium
Curried Tuna Salad								
	287	34 g	27 g	6 g	5 g	638 mg	56 mg	123 mg
French bread (30g/1oz)								
	78	3 g	15 g	1 g	1 g	173 mg	0 mg	21 mg
Vegetable juice (240ml/8fl oz)								
	60	2 g	11 g	0 g	2 g	140 mg	0 mg	40 mg
Vanilla low-fat yogurt (115g/4oz)								
	105	6 g	17 g	1.5 g	0 g	81 mg	6 mg	209 mg
Gingersnaps (3 small)								
	90	1 g	16 g	2 g	0.5 g	128 mg	0 mg	15 mg
Meal Total								
	620	46 g	86 g	10.5 g(15%)	8.5 g	1,160 mg	62 mg	408 mg

Menu
Tomato vegetable soup (ready-made)
Grilled Salmon with Penne Primavera
Mixed Garden Salad
Watermelon wedge

Grilled Salmon with Penne Primavera

SERVES 4   total preparation time: **20 minutes**

225g/8oz penne pasta
4 teaspoons olive oil
4 large cloves garlic, crushed
1 head broccoli, cut into bite-size pieces
2 medium red peppers, cored and cut into 5mm/¼ inch-wide strips
8 large button mushrooms, thinly sliced
1 large onion, halved and thinly sliced
Nonstick cooking spray
125ml/4fl oz lemon juice
Four 170g/6oz salmon steaks or 680g/1½lb salmon fillet
45g/¾oz grated Parmesan cheese

1. Bring 1.5 litres/2½ pints water to the boil in a large pot. Add penne, stir occasionally, and cook 7–8 minutes or until al dente. Drain, set aside and keep warm.
2. Meanwhile, heat 2 teaspoons oil in nonstick frying pan over medium-high heat. Add garlic and sauté until golden, about 30 seconds. Add broccoli, peppers, mushrooms and onion and sauté until tender, 5–7 minutes.
3. Preheat grill. Spray grill pan with cooking spray and place salmon on it.

4. In a small bowl, combine remaining olive oil with lemon juice. Brush on salmon, basting both sides. Grill 3–4 minutes on one side, turn and grill 3–4 minutes more or until fish flakes easily with a fork. Place on plate and keep warm.
5. In a large bowl, combine vegetable mixture with penne. Toss with grated Parmesan cheese. Serve immediately with salmon.

Mixed Garden Salad

SERVES 4   total preparation time: **10–12 minutes**

1 small head round or red-leaf lettuce, torn into bite-size pieces
285g/10oz rocket, tough ends removed
1 small red onion, thinly sliced
24 cherry tomatoes, halved
125ml/4fl oz fat-free salad dressing

Place lettuce in large salad bowl and toss with rocket, onion and tomatoes. Dress immediately before serving.

nutritional information per serving

	Calories	Protein	Carbs	Fat	Fibre	Sodium	Cholesterol	Calcium
Tomato vegetable soup (250ml/8fl oz)								
	80	6 g	17 g	0 g	5 g	240 mg	0 mg	40 mg
Grilled Salmon with Penne Primavera								
	503	42 g	29 g	24 g	4 g	208 mg	98 mg	151 mg
Mixed Garden Salad								
	74	3 g	16 g	1 g	4 g	37 mg	0 mg	56 mg
Watermelon wedge (¹⁄₁₆ melon)								
	92	2 g	21 g	1 g	1 g	6 mg	0 mg	23 mg
Meal Total								
	749	53 g	83 g	26 g (31%)	14 g	491 mg	98 mg	270 mg

Seafood Strata
Asparagus Spears (page 214)
Parsley Carrot Coins (page 137)
Fresh Cooked Beetroot (page 215)
Multicoloured Salad (page 205)
Fresh sweet cherries

Seafood Strata

SERVES 4   total preparation time: **95 minutes (see Note)**

4 slices day-old white bread

Nonstick cooking spray

½ teaspoon olive or rapeseed oil

115g/4oz button mushrooms, thinly sliced

1 spring onion, diced

60ml/2fl oz dry sherry

225g/8oz frozen pollock, defrosted and flaked (substitute cod if pollock
   is unavailable)

55g/2oz reduced-fat Swiss (or alternatively Cheddar) cheese

1 large egg

200ml/7fl oz skimmed milk

⅛ teaspoon salt

⅛ teaspoon ground white pepper

1 large tomato, thinly sliced

1 tablespoon chopped fresh chives

1. Preheat oven to 190°C/375°F/Gas mark 5.
2. Trim crusts from bread, place on ungreased baking sheet and bake 10 minutes, until lightly browned. Reduce heat to 180°C/350°F/Gas mark 4.
3. Spray a large nonstick frying pan with cooking spray, brush with oil and set over medium-high heat. Add mushrooms and sauté 10 minutes, turning occasionally, until liquid has evaporated. Add spring onion and sauté 1–2 minutes. Add sherry, bring to the boil and cook 1 minute. Reduce heat to low, add flaked fish, mix well and remove from heat; set aside.
4. Spray a 20cm/8 inch square glass or ceramic baking dish with vegetable cooking spray. Cut 2 slices of the toasted bread into squares and place in the bottom of the dish. Sprinkle with half the cheese and top with the fish mixture. Cut the remaining 2 slices of bread into squares, distribute over the fish mixture and sprinkle with the remaining cheese.
5. In a large bowl, beat the egg with milk, salt and pepper. Pour egg mixture over top of bread, distributing evenly. Top with tomato slices.
6. Bake 40–45 minutes, or until knife inserted in centre comes out clean. Allow to stand 5 minutes. Garnish with chopped chives and serve.

Note: This strata can be assembled the day before, refrigerated and baked the next day.

nutritional information per serving

	Calories	Protein	Carbs	Fat	Fibre	Sodium	Cholesterol	Calcium
Seafood Strata								
	295	22 g	24 g	11 g	1 g	456 mg	84 mg	349 mg
Asparagus Spears								
	39	4 g	8 g	0.5 g	3.5 g	3 mg	0 mg	36 mg
Parsley Carrot Coins								
	49	1 g	12 g	0 g	3 g	41 mg	0 mg	33 mg
Freshly Cooked Beetroot								
	75	3 g	17 g	0 g	1 g	122 mg	0 mg	27 mg
Multicoloured Salad								
	85	3 g	18 g	1 g	3 g	78 mg	0 mg	127 mg
Fresh sweet cherries (about 12)								
	59	1 g	14 g	1 g	2 g	0 mg	0 mg	12 mg
Meal Total								
	602	34 g	93 g	13.5 g (20%)	14 g	700 mg	84 mg	584 mg

Menu
Grilled Red Snapper with Charred Tomato Salsa
White Rice (page 211)
Tarragon-Scented Broccoli and Cauliflower
Tossed Salad with Walnut Dressing
Fresh plums

Grilled Red Snapper with Charred Tomato Salsa

SERVES 4   **total preparation time: 15 minutes**

Nonstick cooking spray
780g/1¾ lb red snapper fillet (substitute mullet, tuna, or other firm fish)
1 medium red onion, finely diced
4 medium green chillies, cored, seeded and chopped
4 medium tomatoes, halved
2 tablespoons chopped fresh coriander

1. Preheat grill to medium and spray grill pan lightly with cooking spray.
2. Rinse fish and pat dry.
3. In a small bowl, combine onion and chillies. Mix well.
4. Place fish and tomatoes on grill pan. Cook tomatoes 5–6 minutes, until just tender and slightly blackened; remove and set aside. Cook fish 8–10 minutes, or until fish flakes easily with a fork, turning once.
5. While fish is cooking, coarsely chop the tomato and add to onion mixture. Add coriander and toss. Spoon mixture over fish and serve.

Tarragon-Scented Broccoli and Cauliflower

SERVES 4   **total preparation time: 12 minutes**

2 tablespoons chopped fresh tarragon or 2 teaspoons dried
450g/1lb broccoli, cut into florets
450g/1lb cauliflower, cut into florets
1 teaspoon olive oil

1. Fill a large saucepan with 5cm/2 inches water and bring to the boil.
2. Add chopped tarragon to water and reduce heat to simmer. Place broccoli and cauliflower in a steamer or colander over water and steam 5 minutes, or until crisp-tender. Toss with olive oil and serve.

Tossed Salad with Walnut Dressing

SERVES 4   **total preparation time: 10 minutes**

2 little gem lettuces, torn into bite-size pieces

1 small head iceberg lettuce, torn into bite-size pieces

30g/1oz chopped walnuts

60ml/2fl oz raspberry vinegar

2 teaspoons olive oil

2 cloves garlic, crushed

1. Place greens and walnuts in a large salad bowl and toss.
2. In a small screw-top jar, combine vinegar, oil and garlic. Shake well.
3. Dress immediately before serving.

nutritional information per serving

	Calories	Protein	Carbs	Fat	Fibre	Sodium	Cholesterol	Calcium
Grilled Red Snapper with Charred Tomato Salsa								
	265	43 g	15 g	3 g	3 g	148 mg	73 mg	87 mg
White Rice								
	105	29 g	23 g	0.4 g	0.5 g	0 mg	0 mg	3 mg
Tossed Salad with Walnut Dressing								
	110	3 g	10 g	7 g	3 g	33 mg	0 mg	48 mg
Tarragon-Scented Broccoli and Cauliflower								
	71	6 g	12 g	2 g	6 g	65 mg	0 mg	48 mg
Fresh plums (2 medium)								
	72	1 g	17 g	1 g	2 g	0 mg	0 mg	5 mg
Meal Total								
	623	55 g	77 g	13 g (19%)	14.5 g	246 mg	73 mg	143 mg

Herb-Rubbed Grilled Tuna
Corn on the Cob
Grilled Courgettes (page 207)
Steamed Green Beans (page 212)
Chopped Tomato-Cucumber Salad (page 173)
Raspberry sorbet

Herb-Rubbed Grilled Tuna

SERVES 4   **total preparation time: 30 minutes**

1 tablespoon chopped fresh basil

1 tablespoon chopped fresh mint

1 clove garlic, crushed

1 tablespoon lemon juice

1 teaspoon olive oil

780g/1¾ lb fresh tuna fillet (substitute salmon, halibut, swordfish,
     or other firm fillet)

Nonstick cooking spray

1. Place basil, mint, garlic, lemon juice and olive oil in a food
   processor or blender and process until it forms a paste.
2. Wash tuna and pat dry. Spread paste on the tuna, cover and
   refrigerate 15 minutes.
3. Preheat grill.
4. Place tuna on grill pan and cook 5 minutes per side, until centre
   of fish is translucent.

Corn on the Cob

SERVES 4   total preparation time: **8 minutes**

4 small ears corn, husked (outer leaves and silk removed)

1. Fill large covered saucepan with 5cm/2 inches water and bring to the boil.
2. Place corn in boiling water, cover, return to boiling, then reduce heat to low. Simmer 5–6 minutes, or until tender. Do not over-cook.

nutritional information per serving

	Calories	Protein	Carbs	Fat	Fibre	Sodium	Cholesterol	Calcium
Herb-Rubbed Tuna								
	217	44 g	1 g	3 g	0 g	74 mg	93 mg	61 mg
Corn on the Cob								
	83	3 g	19 g	1 g	2 g	13 mg	0 mg	2 mg
Grilled Courgettes								
	47	2 g	11 g	0 g	2 g	16 mg	0 mg	29 mg
Steamed Green Beans								
	35	2 g	8 g	0 g	4 g	7 mg	0 mg	42 mg
Tomato-Cucumber Salad								
	118	5 g	19 g	4 g	6 g	40 mg	2 mg	87 mg
Raspberry sorbet (½ cup)								
	70	1 g	17 g	0 g	0 g	46 mg	0 mg	2 mg
Meal Total								
	570	57 g	75 g	8 g (13%)	14 g	196 mg	95 mg	223 mg

Menu
Grilled Halibut Steak
Fennel-Onion Salad
Tomato Crostini
Steamed Spinach (page 136)
Mixed Berry Compote

Grilled Halibut Steak

SERVES 4   total preparation time: **25 minutes**

Nonstick cooking spray
125ml/4fl oz fat-free vinaigrette dressing
1⅓ tablespoons lemon juice
4 cloves garlic, crushed
Four 200g/7oz halibut steaks, about 2cm/¾ inch thick

1. Preheat grill and lightly coat grill rack with cooking spray.
2. In a shallow glass dish, combine the vinaigrette, lemon juice and garlic. Add halibut steaks and turn to coat. Cover and marinate in refrigerator 15 minutes.
3. Grill fish 4–6 inches from heat, turning once, about 7 minutes total, or until lightly translucent; cut fish in centre to check it is cooked through.

Fennel-Onion Salad

60ml/2fl oz balsamic vinegar

1⅓ tablespoons granulated sugar

2 small heads red-leaf lettuce, torn into bite-size pieces

2 heads fennel, trimmed and thinly sliced

1 small red onion, thinly sliced

1. In a small jar, combine vinegar and sugar. Shake well and set aside.
2. In a large bowl, combine lettuce, sliced fennel and onion. Dress immediately before serving.

Tomato Crostini

½ loaf French bread, cut into eight 2.5cm/1 inch slices

2 large tomatoes, peeled and chopped

1⅓ tablespoons olive oil

1 tablespoon oregano

1. Preheat grill.
2. Place bread on baking sheet and grill 1–2 minutes on each side until golden brown.
3. Meanwhile, combine tomatoes, oil and seasoning in a small bowl. Spread mixture onto each slice of toasted bread.

Mixed Berry Compote

SERVES 4   total preparation time: **10 minutes**

225g/8oz strawberries, hulled and sliced
225g/8oz blueberries
115g/4oz raspberries
4 tablespoons light, low-fat cream-style topping

Combine berries in a large mixing bowl and toss gently. Divide among 4 bowls, drizzle each with 1 tablespoon cream-style topping and chill before serving.

nutritional information per serving

	Calories	Protein	Carbs	Fat	Fibre	Sodium	Cholesterol	Calcium
Grilled Halibut								
	244	42 g	6 g	5 g	0 g	115 mg	64 mg	108 mg
Fennel-Onion Salad								
	74	3 g	17 g	0.5 g	4 g	54 mg	0 mg	79 mg
Tomato Crostini								
	197	5 g	30 g	6 g	3 g	311 mg	0 mg	59 mg
Steamed Spinach								
	36	5 g	6 g	0.5 g	4 g	129 mg	0 mg	162 mg
Mixed Berry Compote								
	92	2 g	27 g	1.5 g	10 g	2 mg	0 mg	33 mg
Meal Total								
	643	57 g	86 g	13.5 g (19%)	21 g	611 mg	64 mg	441 mg

Menu
Lemon-Pepper Sole
Cinnamon-Dusted Sweet Potatoes
Steamed Spinach (page 136)
Oregano-Scented Summer Squash (page 136)
Tossed Salad with Tomatoes (page 132)
Fresh pear

Lemon-Pepper Sole

SERVES 4   **total preparation time: 12–15 minutes**

Nonstick cooking spray
780g/1¾ lb skinless sole fillets, divided into 170–200g/6–7oz portions
1 tablespoon olive oil
1 teaspoon lemon juice
½ teaspoon freshly ground black pepper
4 medium tomatoes, sliced
2 medium spring onions, chopped
½ teaspoon dried basil

1. Preheat grill, and spray rectangular baking dish with cooking spray.
2. Wash fish and pat dry. Brush fish with olive oil and lemon juice, then sprinkle with pepper. Place tomato slices on top of fish and sprinkle with chopped spring onion and basil.
3. Grill 5–7 minutes, or until fish flakes easily.

Cinnamon-Dusted Sweet Potatoes

SERVES 4   total preparation time: **10–15 or 60–70 minutes, depending on method**

2 large sweet potatoes, with skin (see Note), scrubbed well and ends
   trimmed
1 teaspoon ground cinnamon

Oven method: Preheat oven to 200°C/400°F/Gas mark 6. Prick potatoes a few times with a fork. Place on baking sheet and bake 50–60 minutes, or until soft when pierced with a fork. Allow to cool slightly before serving, 5–10 minutes. Split potatoes open and sprinkle with ground cinnamon. *Microwave method:* Prick potatoes twice with a fork. Place side by side in centre of microwave oven. Cook on high 5–8 minutes, or until soft when pierced with a fork. Sprinkle with ground cinnamon.

Note: The skin of sweet potatoes contains lots of nutrients and fibre and should be left on and eaten whenever possible.

nutritional information per serving

	Calories	Protein	Carbs	Fat	Fibre	Sodium	Cholesterol	Calcium
Lemon-Pepper Sole								
	242	39 g	7 g	6 g	2 g	174 mg	95 mg	56 mg
Cinnamon-Dusted Sweet Potatoes								
	99	2 g	25 g	0 g	3 g	34 mg	0 mg	22 mg
Steamed Spinach								
	36	5 g	6 g	0.5 g	4 g	129 mg	0 mg	162 mg
Oregano-Scented Summer Squash								
	23	1 g	5 g	0 g	2 g	2 mg	0 mg	27 mg
Tossed Salad with Tomatoes								
	70	3 g	15 g	1 g	4 g	38 mg	0 mg	52 mg
Fresh pear (1 medium)								
	98	1 g	25 g	1 g	4 g	0 mg	0 mg	18 mg
Meal Total								
	568	51 g	83 g	8.5 g (13%)	19 g	377 mg	95 mg	337 mg

Vegetarian and Soya

Cannellini Bean and Tomato Salad

•

Tofu Vegetable Salad

•

Stuffed Potato Olé

•

Polenta with Grilled Vegetables

•

Penne with Greens and White Beans

•

Spaghetti and Courgettes with Tofu Marinara

•

Vegetable Tofu Lasagne

•

Tempeh with Saucy Green Beans and White Rice

•

Veggie Tofu Stir-Fry with Sesame Seeds and Brown Rice

•

Baked Aubergine Parmesan

•

Quick Tortilla Pizza

•

Easy Bean Burrito

•

Vegetarian Chilli

•

Savoury Baked Soya Beans

•

Tofu Cassoulet

Menu
Low-fat broccoli soup (ready-made)
Cannellini Bean and Tomato Salad
Wholemeal bread
Virtually fat-free strawberry yogurt (artificially sweetened)

Cannellini Bean and Tomato Salad

SERVES 4   **total preparation time: 75 minutes**

1 tablespoon white vinegar

1 tablespoon lemon juice

1 teaspoon Dijon mustard

1 drop liquid hot-pepper seasoning

2 teaspoons olive oil

410g can cannellini beans, drained

½ tablespoon chopped fresh basil

½ tablespoon chopped fresh mint

1 tablespoon chopped fresh parsley

1 spring onion, chopped

1 small clove garlic, crushed

6 cherry tomatoes, halved

½ large red pepper, cored and finely diced

1. In a small bowl, combine vinegar, lemon juice, mustard and hot-pepper seasoning. Beating with a whisk or fork, slowly add the olive oil. Set aside.

2. In a large bowl, combine the drained beans with the basil, mint, parsley, spring onion and garlic. Mix in the dressing, cover and refrigerate at least 15 minutes or up to 4 hours. Immediately before serving, lightly mix in tomatoes and red pepper.

nutritional information per serving

	Calories	Protein	Carbs	Fat	Fibre	Sodium	Cholesterol	Calcium
Cannellini Bean and Tomato Salad								
	166	9 g	28 g	3 g	6 g	189 mg	0 mg	94 mg
Low-fat cream of broccoli soup (240ml/8fl oz)								
	88	2 g	13 g	3 g	2 g	578 mg	5 mg	41 mg
Wholemeal bread (1 slice)								
	69	3 g	13 g	1 g	2 g	148 mg	0 mg	20 mg
Virtually fat-free strawberry yogurt (225g/8oz)								
	90	8 g	14 g	0 g	2 g	140 mg	5 mg	250 mg
Meal Total								
	413	22 g	68 g	7 g (15%)	12 g	1,055 mg	10 mg	405 mg

Lentil and vegetable soup (ready-made)
Tofu Vegetable Salad
French roll
Honeydew melon wedge

Tofu Vegetable Salad

SERVES 4   **total preparation time: 35 minutes**

450g/1lb tofu, cut into small cubes
1 head round lettuce, leaves separated
2 large carrots, grated
2 medium red peppers, cored and cut into strips
2 celery sticks, diced
115g/4oz alfalfa sprouts
2 large cucumbers, peeled and thinly sliced
½ medium red onion, thinly sliced
24 cherry tomatoes, halved
55g/2oz reduced fat Cheddar cheese, grated
30g/1oz sunflower seeds
1 tablespoon olive oil
125ml/4fl oz balsamic vinegar

1. Preheat oven to 180°C/350°F/Gas mark 4.
2. Place tofu in a colander and drain for 10 minutes. Pat dry with kitchen paper. Place on a baking sheet and bake for 20 minutes. Remove and allow to cool.

3. Arrange lettuce leaves on a large serving plate and place baked tofu in centre. Arrange grated carrots, pepper strips, diced celery, sprouts, sliced cucumbers, sliced onion, halved cherry tomatoes and grated cheese around the tofu. Sprinkle sunflower seeds on top. Dress with oil and vinegar immediately before serving.

nutritional information per serving

	Calories	Protein	Carbs	Fat	Fibre	Sodium	Cholesterol	Calcium
Tofu Vegetable Salad								
	265	18 g	25 g	15 g	7 g	265 mg	0 mg	275 mg
Lentil and vegetable soup (250ml/8fl oz)								
	90	6 g	19 g	0 g	4 g	210 mg	0 mg	40 mg
French roll (30g/1oz)								
	79	2 g	14 g	1 g	1 g	173 mg	0 mg	26 mg
Honeydew wedge (⅛ melon)								
	56	1 g	15 g	0 g	1 g	16 mg	0 mg	10 mg
Meal Total								
	490	27 g	73 g	16 g (23%)	13 g	664 mg	0 mg	351 mg

Menu

Easy Minestrone Soup
Stuffed Potato Olé
Chopped Tomato-Cucumber Salad
Tangerines

Easy Minestrone Soup

SERVES 4   **total preparation time: 20 minutes**

1 tablespoon olive oil
½ medium onion, finely diced
1 clove garlic, crushed
1 celery stick, finely diced
450ml/16fl oz low-fat low-sodium vegetable stock
410g can kidney beans
285g/10oz frozen mixed vegetables
1 medium floury potato, peeled and diced
¼ teaspoon dried basil
⅛ teaspoon ground black pepper

1. Heat oil in a large saucepan over medium heat. Add onions, garlic and celery and sauté 3–4 minutes, until onion softens.
2. Add stock, beans, vegetables, potatoes, basil and pepper. Bring to the boil, then reduce heat to low and simmer 15 minutes. Serve warm.

Stuffed Potato Olé

SERVES 4   total preparation time: **15 or 60–70 minutes, depending on method**

4 medium baking potatoes, well-scrubbed
225g/8oz reduced-fat mature Cheddar cheese, grated
4 tablespoons very low fat natural yogurt
1 red pepper, cored and finely diced
4 tablespoons chopped chives

1. Bake potato. *Oven method:* Preheat oven to 200°C/400°F/Gas mark 6. Prick each potato a few times with a fork, place on baking sheet and cook 50–60 minutes, or until soft when pricked with a fork. *Microwave method:* Prick each potato a few times with a fork, place side by side in centre of microwave oven and cook on high 5–8 minutes, or until soft when pricked with a fork.
2. Preheat grill. Split baked potatoes and top with grated cheese. Place potatoes on a tray and grill until cheese begins to melt, 4–5 minutes. Remove from grill and top with yogurt, diced pepper and chopped chives.

Chopped Tomato-Cucumber Salad

SERVES 4   total preparation time: **10 minutes**

1 small head iceberg lettuce, torn into bite-size pieces
1 small head red-leaf lettuce, torn into bite-size pieces
4 large cucumbers, peeled and thinly sliced
4 medium tomatoes, quartered
125ml/4fl oz fat-free dressing

Place greens in a large salad bowl and toss with cucumbers and tomatoes. Dress immediately before serving.

nutritional information per serving

	Calories	Protein	Carbs	Fat	Fibre	Sodium	Cholesterol	Calcium
Easy Minestrone Soup								
	224	10 g	37 g	5 g	8 g	483 mg	2 mg	68 mg
Stuffed Potato Olé								
	313	22 g	36 g	9 g	3 g	218 mg	30 mg	550 mg
Tomato- Cucumber Salad								
	118	5 g	19 g	4 g	6 g	40 mg	2 mg	87 mg
Tangerines (2 small)								
	74	1 g	19 g	0 g	4 g	2 mg	0 mg	24 mg
Meal Total								
	729	38 g	111 g	18 g (22%)	21 g	743 mg	34 mg	729 mg

Menu

Tomato juice with a squeeze of lemon juice
Polenta with Grilled Vegetables
Tossed Salad with Sprouts, Seeds and Beans
Frozen low-fat yogurt

Polenta with Grilled Vegetables

SERVES 4   **total preparation time: 25 minutes**

130g/4½oz polenta (ground cornmeal)
4 teaspoons olive oil
60ml/2fl oz balsamic vinegar
4 tablespoons chopped fresh basil
4 cloves garlic, crushed
¼ teaspoon ground pepper
2 yellow peppers, cored and sliced
4 medium onions, quartered
4 tomatoes, quartered
6 large mushrooms, halved

1. Preheat grill.
2. In a large bowl, combine cornmeal with 250ml/8fl oz cold water. Stir to mix. Bring 750ml/25fl oz water to the boil in a medium saucepan. When water begins to boil, *gradually* stir in cornmeal mixture. Reduce heat immediately to low, cover and steam 15 minutes, stirring frequently.
3. Meanwhile, combine olive oil, vinegar, basil, garlic and pepper in a large mixing bowl. Add the vegetables and toss well to coat.
4. Place vegetables on a baking sheet or grill pan. Grill under high heat until al dente, about 8–10 minutes. Do not overcook.
5. Top cooked polenta with vegetables and serve.

Tossed Salad
with Sprouts, Seeds and Beans

SERVES 4   total preparation time: **10 minutes**

1 head round lettuce, torn into bite-size pieces
1 small head iceberg lettuce, torn into bite-size pieces
24 cherry tomatoes, washed and halved
55g/2oz alfalfa sprouts
410g can kidney beans, drained
125ml/4fl oz fat-free salad dressing
4 tablespoons sunflower seeds

In a large salad bowl, toss lettuce with tomatoes, sprouts and kidney beans. Immediately before serving, dress, divide evenly among 4 salad plates and top each with 1 tablespoon sunflower seeds.

nutritional information per serving

	Calories	Protein	Carbs	Fat	Fibre	Sodium	Cholesterol	Calcium
Tomato juice cocktail with lemon juice (250ml/8fl oz)								
	60	2 g	11 g	0 g	2 g	140 mg	0 mg	40 mg
Polenta								
	190	5 g	39 g	1 g	2 g	1 mg	0 mg	2 mg
Grilled Vegetables								
	137	4 g	21 g	5.5 g	4 g	20 mg	0 mg	44 mg
Tossed Salad with Sprouts, Seeds and Beans								
	201	11 g	31 g	5 g	8 g	404 mg	0 mg	102 mg
Frozen low-fat yogurt (115g/4oz)								
	95	5 g	19 g	2 g	0 g	64 mg	2 mg	167 mg
Meal Total								
	683	27 g	121 g	13.5 g (18%)	16 g	629 mg	2 mg	355 mg

Penne with Greens and White Beans
Asparagus Spears (page 214)
Tomato, Egg and Cucumber Salad
Strawberries

Penne with Greens and White Beans

SERVES 4   total preparation time: **25 minutes**

4 teaspoons olive oil

4 cloves garlic, crushed

1 medium red pepper, cored and diced

900g/2lb fresh greens (spinach, kale or Swiss chard), stems removed,
    and torn into bite-size pieces

4 teaspoons balsamic vinegar

125ml/4fl oz vegetable stock

Two 410g cans cannellini or other white beans, drained

225g/8oz penne pasta

4 tablespoons grated Parmesan cheese

1. Bring a large pan of water to the boil for the pasta.
2. Heat the oil in a large nonstick frying pan over medium-high
    heat. Add garlic and pepper, and sauté 2 minutes. Stir in greens, vin-
    egar and stock, cover pan and cook until greens are wilted and
    tender but still bright green, 5–7 minutes. Gently stir the beans
    into greens mixture, set aside and keep warm until pasta is ready.
3. Meanwhile, cook pasta according to package directions, until al
    dente. Drain.
4. Add pasta to bean mixture and gently mix. Top each serving with
    1 tablespoon grated Parmesan.

Tomato, Egg and Cucumber Salad

SERVES 4   **total preparation time: 15 minutes**

4 large eggs
125ml/4fl oz balsamic vinegar
4 teaspoons olive oil
4 medium tomatoes, cut into 5mm/¼ inch slices
2 large cucumbers, peeled and thinly sliced
½ head red or green lettuce, separated into leaves

1. Place eggs in a saucepan with water to cover at least 2.5cm/
   1 inch above eggs, and bring to the boil. Immediately after water
   has boiled, reduce heat to just below simmering, cover and cook
   eggs 15–20 minutes. Cool at once in cold water (this prevents the
   yolk from darkening and makes for easier peeling). Once cool,
   peel and slice into 5mm/¼ inch slices.
2. Meanwhile, combine vinegar and oil in screw-top jar; shake well.
3. Toss tomatoes, cucumbers and lettuce in a large salad bowl.
   Immediately before serving, toss with dressing, then top with
   sliced egg.

nutritional information per serving

	Calories	Protein	Carbs	Fat	Fibre	Sodium	Cholesterol	Calcium
Penne with Greens and White Beans								
	520	26 g	85 g	9 g	14 g	839 mg	5 mg	409 mg
Asparagus Spears								
	39	4 g	8 g	0.5 g	3.5 g	3 mg	0 mg	36 mg
Tomato, Egg and Cucumber Salad								
	190	9 g	16 g	11 g	3 g	90 mg	212 mg	73 mg
Strawberries								
	50	1 g	12 g	0.6 g	4 g	2 mg	0 mg	23 mg
Meal Total								
	799	40 g	121 g	21.1 g (24%)	24.5 g	934 mg	217 mg	541 mg

Spaghetti and Courgette with Tofu Marinara
Mixed Green Salad
Fat-free pudding

Spaghetti and Courgettes with Tofu Marinara

SERVES 4   total preparation time: **80 minutes**

450g/1lb firm tofu
225g/8oz spaghetti
1 tablespoon olive oil
1 medium onion, thinly sliced
4 cloves garlic, crushed
2 medium courgettes, cut into 5mm/¼ inch slices
4 medium tomatoes, diced
225g/8oz tomato passata
1 bay leaf
¼ teaspoon ground black pepper
¼ teaspoon dried basil
¼ teaspoon dried oregano
20g/¾oz grated Parmesan cheese

1. Break tofu into coarse chunks and drain in a colander 10 minutes. Wrap in kitchen paper for 20 minutes.
2. Meanwhile, bring a large pan of water to the boil. Cook spaghetti according to package directions until al dente, 10–12 minutes. Remove from heat, drain, set aside in a large serving bowl and keep warm.
3. Meanwhile, spread oil in a large nonstick pan and set over

medium-high heat. Add onion and garlic and sauté until onions are translucent, 3–4 minutes. Add courgettes and tofu and sauté 5–10 minutes until tofu browns. Add tomatoes, passata, bay leaf, pepper, basil and oregano and reduce heat to low. Cover and simmer 15 minutes. Uncover and simmer an additional 10 minutes. Remove and discard bay leaf.

4. Pour the cooked sauce over the cooked spaghetti and top with grated Parmesan.

Mixed Green Salad

SERVES 4   **total preparation time: 10 minutes**

1 small head red- or green-leaf lettuce, torn into bite-size pieces
1 small head cos lettuce, torn into bite-size pieces
12 very fresh button mushrooms, thinly sliced
2 medium red peppers, cored and diced
4 medium tomatoes, quartered
125ml/4fl oz fat-free salad dressing

Toss all ingredients except dressing in a large salad bowl. Dress immediately before serving.

nutritional information per serving

	Calories	Protein	Carbs	Fat	Fibre	Sodium	Cholesterol	Calcium
Spaghetti and Courgette with Tofu Marinara								
	381	20 g	55 g	11 g	9 g	167 mg	5 mg	297 mg
Mixed Green Salad								
	115	6 g	24 g	1 g	7 g	44 mg	0 mg	131 mg
Fat-free pudding (115g/4oz)								
	100	2 g	23 g	0 g	0 g	241 mg	0 mg	80 mg
Meal Total								
	596	28 g	102 g	12 g (18%)	16 g	452 mg	5 mg	508 mg

Vegetable Tofu Lasagne
Tossed Salad (page 175)
Italian bread
Sliced kiwi fruit

Vegetable Tofu Lasagne

SERVES 6   total preparation time: **2 hours**

450g/1lb firm tofu

225g/8oz dry lasagne sheets

1 tablespoon olive oil

3 cloves garlic, crushed

½ small onion, finely diced

450g/1lb button mushrooms, thinly sliced

1 teaspoon dried basil

1 teaspoon dried oregano

Two 400g cans tomato passata

200g jar tomato purée

450g/1lb fresh spinach, ends removed, and chopped

450g/1lb carrots, trimmed and grated

450g/1lb courgettes, trimmed, and grated

225g/8oz virtually fat-free fromage frais

20g/¾oz grated Parmesan cheese

1. Preheat oven to 200°C/400°F/Gas mark 6, and bring a large saucepan of water to the boil.

2. Break tofu into coarse chunks and drain in a colander 10 minutes. Remove and wrap in kitchen paper for 20 minutes to remove excess moisture. Set aside.

3. Add lasagne sheets to boiling water and cook according to package directions until al dente; do not overcook. Drain, set aside and keep warm. (If you prefer, use the sheets that require no pre-cooking.)

4. Meanwhile, heat oil over medium-high heat in a large frying pan. Add drained tofu, garlic, onions, mushrooms, basil and oregano. Cook, stirring often, until onions are soft and liquid has evaporated, 6–7 minutes. Add passata and tomato purée, heat for a few moments, stirring to blend; set aside.

5. In a large bowl, mix spinach, carrots and courgettes with the cheese.

6. Assemble the lasagne in a 22 x 32cm/9 x 13 inch baking dish: spread a third of the tomato sauce on bottom of pan and arrange half the pasta sheets, overlapping slightly, on top of the sauce. Spread half of the vegetable and cheese mixture on top of the pasta. Repeat with another layer of sauce, pasta and vegetable mixture. Top with the remaining sauce and sprinkle with the grated Parmesan.

7. Bake, uncovered, until hot in the centre, 25–30 minutes. Allow to stand 10 minutes before serving.

nutritional information per serving

	Calories	Protein	Carbs	Fat	Fibre	Sodium	Cholesterol	Calcium
Vegetable Tofu Lasagne								
	457	27 g	62 g	14 g	10 g	306 mg	26 mg	511 mg
Tossed Salad								
	88	5 g	18 g	1 g	5 g	35 mg	0 mg	73 mg
Italian bread								
	77	2.5 g	14 g	1 g	1 g	165 mg	0 mg	22 mg
Sliced kiwi fruit (1)								
	50	1 g	12 g	0.5 g	2 g	0 mg	0 mg	30 mg
Meal Total								
	672	35.5 g	106 g	16.5 g (22%)	18 g	506 mg	26 mg	636 mg

Menu

Tempeh with Saucy Green Beans and Rice
Five-Veggie Salad
Banana

Tempeh with
Saucy Green Beans and Rice

SERVES 4   total preparation time: **55 minutes**

200g/7oz uncooked white rice
Two 225g/8oz cakes tempeh (substitute firm tofu if necessary)
3 tablespoons tamari
1 tablespoon sesame oil
½ medium onion, finely diced
3 large cloves garlic, crushed
1 red chilli pepper, cored and finely diced
225g/8oz tomato passata
115g/4oz tomato purée
450g/1lb green beans, trimmed

1. Place rice and 500ml/18fl oz water in medium saucepan. Cover and bring to the boil. Reduce heat to low and simmer 15–20 minutes, or until all the water is absorbed.
2. Cut tempeh in half widthways, then cut into strips (similar to bacon). Place in a shallow dish with tamari, cover and refrigerate 15 minutes, turning once.

3. Meanwhile, add oil to a wok or large nonstick frying pan and heat over medium-high heat. Add onion, garlic and chilli pepper and stir-fry until onions soften a little, 2–3 minutes. Drain tempeh, add to wok and stir-fry 5–7 minutes, until golden brown. Add passata, tomato purée and green beans, bring almost to boiling, then immediately reduce heat to low, cover and simmer 10 minutes. Serve immediately with the cooked white rice.

Five-Veggie Salad

SERVES 4   **total preparation time: 10 minutes**

2 large tomatoes, quartered and thinly sliced
1 large cucumber, peeled and thinly sliced
2 celery sticks, diced
2 large carrots, grated
6 radishes, sliced
1 tablespoon chopped parsley
2 tablespoons lemon juice
1 tablespoon olive oil
1 clove garlic, crushed

1. In a large bowl, toss tomatoes, cucumber, celery, carrots, radishes and parsley.
2. In a small screw-top jar, combine lemon juice, olive oil and garlic. Shake well.
3. Dress salad immediately before serving.

nutritional information per serving

	Calories	Protein	Carbs	Fat	Fibre	Sodium	Cholesterol	Calcium
Tempeh with Saucy Green Beans and Rice								
	531	31 g	80 g	13 g	13.5 g	809 mg	0 mg	194 mg
Five-Veggie Salad								
	82	2 g	12 g	3 g	3 g	42 mg	0 mg	37 mg
Banana (1 medium)								
	109	1 g	28 g	1 g	3 g	1 mg	0 mg	7 mg
Meal Total								
	722	34 g	120 g	16.6 g (21%)	19.5 g	852 mg	0 mg	238 mg

Easy Veggie Tofu Stir-Fry with Sesame Seeds and Brown Rice

SERVES 4   **total preparation time: 1 hour**

900g/2lb firm tofu, cut into 2.5cm/1 inch cubes

3 tablespoons light (reduced-sodium) soy sauce

570ml/1 pint vegetable stock or water

140g/5oz brown rice

1 tablespoon rapeseed or olive oil

4 cloves garlic, crushed

1 medium onion, thinly sliced

450g/1lb broccoli, cut into bite-size florets

2 large red peppers, cored and thinly sliced

225g/8oz button mushrooms, thinly sliced

220g can water chestnuts, drained

½ teaspoon dried basil

½ teaspoon dried oregano

½ teaspoon ground black pepper

30g/1oz sesame seeds

1. Place tofu in a colander and drain 10 minutes. Pat dry with kitchen paper. Place soy sauce in a shallow dish, add tofu, cover, refrigerate and marinate 15 minutes, or up to 1 hour, turning once.

2. In medium covered saucepan, bring 500ml/18fl oz vegetable stock or water to the boil. Slowly stir in rice, cover and reduce heat to low. Simmer 40 minutes, or until all the water is absorbed.

3. Meanwhile, heat the oil in a wok, large frying pan, or heavy saucepan over medium-high heat. Add garlic and onion and sauté until onions soften a little, 2–3 minutes. Add broccoli and red peppers, the remaining stock or water and cook, stirring frequently, 5 minutes. Add mushrooms, water chestnuts, basil, oregano and black pepper and continue to cook 2 more minutes, or until mushrooms are soft. Add sesame seeds and the marinated tofu with soy sauce and cook, stirring gently, until tofu is heated through, about 5 minutes. Serve with the cooked rice.

Berry-Peach Salad

SERVES 4   **total preparation time: 10 minutes**

225g/8oz strawberries, hulled and sliced
225g/8oz blueberries, washed, cleaned
4 medium peaches, stoned and sliced
½ teaspoon lemon juice
Artificial sweetener (optional)

In large bowl, combine strawberries, blueberries and peaches with lemon juice. Sprinkle with sugar substitute, if desired. Serve chilled.

nutritional information per serving

	Calories	Protein	Carbs	Fat	Fibre	Sodium	Cholesterol	Calcium
Tomato soup (250ml/8fl oz)								
	99	3 g	19 g	1 g	4 g	480 mg	0 mg	56 mg
Easy Veggie Tofu Stir-Fry with Sesame Seeds and Brown Rice								
	387	20 g	51 g	14 g	8 g	463 mg	0 mg	289 mg
Berry-Peach Salad								
	102	2 g	29 g	0.5 g	7 g	39 mg	0 mg	24 mg
Meal Total								
	588	25 g	99 g	15.5 g (23%)	19 g	982 mg	0 mg	369 mg

Baked Aubergine Parmesan
Multicoloured Salad (page 205)
Fruit salad (ready-made)

Baked Aubergine Parmesan

SERVES 4   total preparation time: **85 minutes**

Nonstick cooking spray
200ml/7fl oz soya milk or skimmed milk
55g/2oz breadcrumbs
85g/3oz wheat germ
1 teaspoon basil
½ teaspoon oregano
½ teaspoon thyme
¼ teaspoon salt
2 medium aubergines, cut into 1cm/½ inch slices
500ml/18fl oz tomato passata
125g pack light mozzarella cheese, thinly sliced
45g/1½oz grated Parmesan cheese

1. Preheat oven to 190°C/375°F/Gas mark 5. Spray nonstick baking sheet with cooking spray.
2. Place milk in shallow bowl.
3. In second bowl, combine breadcrumbs, wheat germ, basil, oregano, thyme and salt.
4. Dip aubergine slices first in milk, then in breadcrumb mixture to coat both sides. Place prepared aubergine slices on baking sheet and bake until tender, about 25–30 minutes. Remove from oven, cover and keep warm.

5. Spread some passata over the bottom of a large casserole dish. Add a layer of aubergine, then more passata. Repeat layers until all the ingredients are used. Spread the mozzarella over the top and sprinkle with Parmesan cheese.

6. Bake, uncovered, in the preheated oven for 45 minutes, or until edges are bubbly. Allow to sit for 10 minutes before cutting. Serve hot.

nutritional information per serving

	Calories	Protein	Carbs	Fat	Fibre	Sodium	Cholesterol	Calcium
Baked Aubergine Parmesan								
	510	39 g	63 g	13 g	14 g	1,085 mg	20 mg	1,109 mg
Multicoloured Salad								
	85	3 g	18 g	1 g	3 g	78 mg	0 mg	127 mg
Fruit salad (225g/8oz)								
	74	1 g	19 g	0 g	2 g	7 mg	0 mg	17 mg
Meal Total								
	669	43 g	100 g	14 g (19%)	19 g	1,170 mg	20 mg	1,253 mg

Menu
Quick Tortilla Pizza
Avocado Salad
Cucumber batons
Fresh sliced strawberries

Quick Tortilla Pizza

SERVES 4   **total preparation time: 15–25 minutes**

4 large flour tortillas (see Note)
410g can low-salt, low-sugar baked beans, drained
2 large tomatoes, washed and chopped
55g/2oz reduced-fat Cheddar cheese, grated
½ head iceberg lettuce, shredded
225g/8oz salsa
12 large pitted black olives, very thinly sliced
55g/2oz very low fat natural yogurt

1. Preheat grill.
2. Place tortillas on a baking sheet. Layer drained beans, tomatoes and cheese evenly among tortillas and grill 2–3 minutes, or until cheese melts.
3. Remove from grill and top each with equal portions of the shredded lettuce, salsa, sliced olives and yogurt.

Note: To warm tortillas in the microwave, place flat in microwave and heat on medium 45–50 seconds until hot; do not overheat. Oven method: Wrap tortillas in aluminium foil and warm in 130°C/250°F/Gas mark ½ oven 10 minutes.

Avocado Salad

SERVES 4 total preparation time: **10–12 minutes**

1 small head iceberg lettuce, torn into bite-size pieces
1 small head red-leaf lettuce, torn into bite-size pieces
1 medium ripe avocado, stoned and diced
1 small red onion, thinly sliced
125ml/4fl oz balsamic vinegar

Place lettuce in a large bowl and toss with diced avocado and sliced onion. Dress with balsamic vinegar immediately before serving.

nutritional information per serving

	Calories	Protein	Carbs	Fat	Fibre	Sodium	Cholesterol	Calcium
Quick Tortilla Pizza								
	395	19 g	63 g	8 g	11 g	1,432 mg	8 mg	289 mg
Avocado Salad								
	127	3 g	13 g	8 g	5 g	27 mg	0 mg	56 mg
Cucumber batons								
	12	0.5 g	3 g	0 g	0.7 g	2 mg	0 mg	14 mg
Fresh sliced strawberries (115g/4oz)								
	50	1 g	12 g	0.6 g	4 g	2 mg	0 mg	23 mg
Meal Total								
	584	23.5 g	91 g	16.6 g (26%)	20.7 g	1,463 mg	8 mg	382 mg

Gazpacho (ready-made)

Easy Bean Burrito

Mandarin oranges

Easy Bean Burrito

SERVES 4   **total preparation time: 15–25 minutes**

1 tablespoon olive oil

4 cloves garlic, crushed

½ medium onion, diced

425g can black beans, drained

Two 195g cans corn kernels, drained

4 medium flour tortillas, warmed (see Note)

115g/4oz reduced-fat mild Cheddar cheese, grated

½ head iceberg lettuce, shredded

1 spring onion, chopped

55g/2oz very low fat natural yogurt

1. Heat oil in a large nonstick frying pan over medium-high heat.
   Add garlic and onion and sauté until golden, 4 minutes. Add
   beans and corn, reduce heat to low and cook until mixture is
   heated through, 4–5 minutes.
2. Lay tortillas on a work surface. Evenly divide the bean mixture
   among the tortillas and top with the grated cheese, shredded lettuce and chopped spring onion. Roll the tortillas and top each
   with 1 tablespoon yogurt.

Note: To warm tortillas in the microwave, place flat in microwave and heat on medium 45–50 seconds until hot; do not overheat. Oven method: Wrap tortillas in aluminium foil and warm in a 130°C/250°F/Gas mark ½ oven 10 minutes.

nutritional information per serving

	Calories	Protein	Carbs	Fat	Fibre	Sodium	Cholesterol	Calcium
Gazpacho (250ml/8fl oz)								
	46	7 g	4 g	0.5 g	0.5 g	739 mg	0 mg	24 mg
Easy Bean Burrito								
	552	28 g	84 g	13.5 g	16 g	439 mg	15 mg	386 mg
Mandarin oranges (115g/4oz)								
	53	1 g	12 g	0 g	0 g	0 mg	0 mg	15 mg
Meal Total								
	651	36 g	100 g	14 g (19%)	16.5 g	1,267 mg	15 mg	458 mg

Vegetarian Chilli with Rice

SERVES 4   total preparation time: **60 minutes**

200g/7oz brown rice
1 tablespoon olive oil
4 small cloves garlic, crushed
1 medium onion, finely diced
2 celery sticks, finely diced
2 large carrots, diced
Two 400g cans chopped tomatoes in juice
285g/10oz canned chickpeas, drained
500g/18oz canned kidney beans, drained
2 teaspoons chilli powder
½ teaspoon ground black pepper
55g/2oz grated reduced-fat medium Cheddar cheese

1. Bring 500ml/18fl oz water to the boil in a medium covered
   saucepan. Slowly stir in rice, cover, reduce heat to low and
   simmer 40 minutes, or until all the water is absorbed.

2. Meanwhile, heat oil in a large, covered saucepan over medium-high heat. Add garlic and sauté until golden, about 30 seconds. Add onions, celery and carrots and sauté, stirring frequently, until onions soften, 3–4 minutes. Stir in tomatoes, chickpeas, kidney beans, chilli powder and black pepper. Increase heat to high and bring to the boil, then reduce heat to low, cover and simmer 10 minutes.

3. Serve with the cooked brown rice, and top each serving with 2 tablespoons grated cheese.

nutritional information per serving

	Calories	Protein	Carbs	Fat	Fibre	Sodium	Cholesterol	Calcium
Vegetarian Chilli with Rice								
	575	26 g	104 g	7 g	19 g	1,200 mg	3 mg	434 mg
Mixed Green Salad								
	115	6 g	24 g	1 g	7 g	44 mg	0 mg	131 mg
Cantaloupe wedge (¼ melon)								
	24	1 g	6 g	0.5 g	0.5 g	6 mg	0 mg	8 mg
Meal Total								
	714	33 g	134 g	8.5 g (10%)	26.5 g	1,250 mg	3 mg	573 mg

Savoury Baked Soya Beans
Tomato, Egg and Cucumber Salad (page 177)
Mixed Berry Compote (page 162)

Savoury Baked Soya Beans

SERVES 4   **total preparation time: 3–4 hours to prepare soya beans, 3 hours to prepare casserole**

310g/12oz cooked soya beans, drained

500ml/18fl oz tomato passata

1 large onion, finely diced

2 cloves garlic, crushed

1 teaspoon dry mustard

2 teaspoons chilli powder

¼ teaspoon ground black pepper

2 tablespoons dark treacle

1. Preheat oven to 150°C/300°F/Gas mark 2.
2. In a large casserole dish, combine 700ml/32fl oz of water with all ingredients. Bake for 3 hours, stirring occasionally. If casserole becomes dry during cooking, add water in small increments. Allow to cool 10 minutes before serving.

nutritional information per serving

	Calories	Protein	Carbs	Fat	Fibre	Sodium	Cholesterol	Calcium
Savoury Baked Soya Beans								
	451	35 g	43 g	19 g	11 g	173 mg	0 mg	330 mg
Tomato, Egg and Cucumber Salad								
	190	9 g	16 g	11 g	3 g	90 mg	212 mg	73 mg
Mixed Berry Compote								
	88	1 g	23 g	1.5 g	7 g	2 mg	0 mg	26 mg
Meal Total								
	733	46 g	86 g	31.5 g (39%)	24 g	265 mg	212 mg	436 mg

Tofu Cassoulet
Mushroom Bouillon
Wild Rice (page 143)
Asparagus Spears (page 214)
Fresh plums

Tofu Cassoulet

SERVES 4   total preparation time: **70 minutes**

450g/1lb firm tofu, cut into 2.5cm/1 inch cubes
Nonstick cooking spray
1 tablespoon olive oil
4 cloves garlic, crushed
2 medium carrots, grated
½ medium onion, finely diced
2 medium tomatoes, chopped
225g/8oz button mushrooms, sliced
450g/1lb fresh spinach, ends removed
¼ teaspoon dried oregano
¼ teaspoon dried basil
¼ teaspoon ground black pepper
410g can cannellini beans, drained
85g/3oz salsa
125g pack light mozzarella cheese, grated

1. Preheat oven to 180°C/350°F/Gas mark 4.
2. Place tofu in a colander and drain for 20 minutes. Pat dry with kitchen paper, crumble into small pieces and set aside.

3. Spray a large nonstick frying pan with vegetable cooking spray. Add half the oil and sauté tofu over medium-high heat until browned, 5–10 minutes. Remove from pan and set aside.

4. Add garlic, carrots, onion and remaining oil to pan and sauté until onion is translucent, 3–4 minutes. Add tomatoes and cook until soft, another 3–4 minutes. Add mushrooms and spinach, and continue cooking until spinach is wilted but still bright green, 2 minutes. Add oregano, basil and pepper. Mix gently and remove from heat.

5. In a large baking dish, layer half the beans, top with half the cooked vegetables, half the salsa, half the tofu and half the mozzarella. Repeat the layers with the other half of the ingredients, ending with cheese on top.

6. Bake for 35 minutes, or until cheese is lightly golden. Allow to cool 10 minutes before serving.

Mushroom Bouillon

SERVES 4   total preparation time: **55 minutes**

200g/7oz button mushrooms, diced (reserve 3 unblemished
    mushrooms for garnish; cut into slices)
1 celery stick, diced
1 small carrot, diced
¼ medium onion, diced
2 tablespoons dry sherry
Freshly ground black pepper
570ml/20fl oz low-sodium beef stock

1. Place mushrooms, celery, carrot, onion and 340ml/12fl oz water
    in a large covered saucepan and bring to the boil. Reduce heat to
    low and simmer, partially covered, 45 minutes. Add sherry and
    pepper and simmer, uncovered, 2 minutes.
2. Strain through a fine-mesh sieve or strainer, pressing vegetables
    to extract as much juice as possible. Add beef stock and simmer
    until heated through. Serve garnished with reserved mushroom
    slices.

nutritional information per serving

	Calories	Protein	Carbs	Fat	Fibre	Sodium	Cholesterol	Calcium
Tofu Cassoulet								
	408	28 g	46 g	15g	12 g	589 mg	16 mg	520 mg
Mushroom Bouillon								
	48	4 g	4.5 g	1 g	1 g	59 mg	0 mg	17 mg
Wild Rice								
	80	3 g	17 g	0 g	1 g	2 mg	0 mg	2 mg
Asparagus Spears								
	39	4 g	8 g	0.5 g	3.5 g	3 mg	0 mg	36 mg
Plums (2 medium)								
	73	1 g	17 g	1 g	2 g	0 mg	0 mg	5 mg
Meal Total								
	648	40 g	92.5 g	17.5 g (24%)	19.5 g	653 mg	16 mg	580 mg

Beef and Lamb

Grilled Sirloin

•

Cajun Grilled Steak

•

Veal Chops with Papaya Salsa

•

Greek-Style Burrito

•

Mint-Glazed Lamb Chop

Menu
Grilled Sirloin
Garlicky Oven Fries
Asparagus Spears (page 214)
Parsley Carrot Coins (page 137)
Multicoloured Salad
Honeydew melon wedge

Grilled Sirloin

SERVES 4   **total preparation time: 15 minutes**

Four 200g/7oz lean sirloin steaks, about 1.5cm/¾ inch thick, trimmed
of fat

1. Preheat grill.
2. Grill steaks, turning once, 4–5 minutes per side, depending on
   thickness and how cooked you like your steak. (To test, cut a slit
   and note colour: pink indicates medium, grey indicates well
   done.) Remove from grill and allow to rest 2–3 minutes before
   serving, for juices to set.

Garlicky Oven Fries

SERVES 4   **total preparation time: 30 minutes**

125ml/4fl oz low-sodium chicken stock

1 teaspoon garlic powder

⅛ teaspoon ground black pepper

4 medium baking potatoes, unpeeled and cut lengthwise into long, thin
    chips

Vegetable cooking spray

1. Preheat oven to 200°C/400°F/Gas mark 6.
2. In a large bowl, combine stock with garlic powder and black
   pepper. Add potato chips and toss to coat well.
3. Spray a baking sheet with vegetable cooking spray. Arrange potatoes in a single layer and bake 20–25 minutes, turning frequently,
   until crisp-tender.

Multicoloured Salad

SERVES 4   **total preparation time: 12 minutes**

225g/8oz radicchio, torn into bite-size pieces

225g/8oz rocket

1 head round lettuce, torn into bite-size pieces

1 head endive, separated into leaves

2 large carrots, cut into 5mm/¼ inch slices

125ml/4fl oz fat-free vinaigrette dressing

Place greens in a large bowl and toss with carrots. Dress with vinaigrette. Serve immediately.

nutritional information per serving

	Calories	Protein	Carbs	Fat	Fibre	Sodium	Cholesterol	Calcium
Grilled Sirloin								
	258	42 g	0 g	9 g	0 g	115 mg	121 mg	14 mg
Garlicky Oven Fries								
	139	3 g	31 g	0.5 g	3 g	23 mg	0 mg	15 mg
Multicoloured Salad								
	85	3 g	18 g	1 g	3 g	78 g	0 mg	127 mg
Asparagus Spears								
	39	4 g	8 g	0.5 g	3.5 g	3 mg	0 mg	36 mg
Parsley Carrot Coins								
	49	1 g	12 g	0 g	3 g	41 mg	0 mg	33 mg
Honeydew melon wedge (⅙ melon)								
	56	1 g	15 g	0 g	1 g	16 mg	0 mg	10 mg
Meal Total								
	626	54 g	84 g	11 g (16%)	13.5 g	276 mg	121 mg	235 mg

Menu

Cajun Grilled Flank Steak

Grilled Courgettes

Small Baked Potato

Corn on the Cob (page 159)

Fennel-Onion Salad (page 161)

Mango

Cajun Grilled Flank Steak

SERVES 4   total preparation time: **45 minutes**

2 teaspoons Cajun seasoning

2 cloves garlic, crushed

2 tablespoons low-sodium beef stock

780g/1¾ lb flank steak (or your favourite lean cut)

1. In a small bowl, combine Cajun seasoning, garlic and beef stock. Rub steak with mixture, cover and refrigerate 20 minutes.
2. Meanwhile, preheat grill. Grill meat, turning once, 4–5 minutes per side, depending on thickness and how cooked you like your steak. (To test, cut a slit and note colour: pink indicates medium, grey indicates well done.)
3. Remove from grill and allow to rest 2–3 minutes, for juices to set. Slice steak thinly across the grain and baste with cooking juices.

Grilled Courgettes

SERVES 4   total preparation time: **10–15 minutes**

4 large courgettes, cut lengthways into 5mm/¼ inch strips
125ml/4fl oz fat-free salad dressing

1. Preheat grill.
2. Brush courgette strips with dressing. Lay strips on grill rack and grill until crisp-tender, 5–10 minutes, turning once.

nutritional information per serving

	Calories	Protein	Carbs	Fat	Fibre	Sodium	Cholesterol	Calcium
Cajun Flank Steak								
	417	54 g	1 g	20 g	0 g	404 mg	133 mg	17 mg
Grilled Courgettes								
	47	2 g	11 g	0 g	2 g	16 mg	0 mg	29 mg
Baked Potato								
	104	2 g	24 g	0 g	2.5 g	49 mg	0 mg	17 mg
Corn on the Cob								
	83	3 g	19 g	1 g	2 g	13 mg	0 mg	2 mg
Fennel-Onion Salad								
	74	3 g	17 g	0.5 g	4 g	54 mg	0 mg	79 mg
Mango (100g/3½ oz)								
	54	0.5 g	14 g	0 g	1.5 g	2 mg	0 mg	8 mg
Meal Total								
	779	64.5 g	86 g	21.5 g (25%)	12 g	538 mg	133 mg	152 mg

Greek-Style Burrito

SERVES 4   total preparation time: **30–40 minutes**

140g/5oz uncooked white rice
780g/1¾ lb extra-lean (91%) minced beef
4 small cloves garlic, crushed
½ teaspoon dried mint
½ teaspoon dried oregano
½ teaspoon cumin
¼ teaspoon salt
55g/2oz natural very low fat yogurt
Four 15cm/6 inch flour tortillas, warmed (see Note)
½ head iceberg lettuce, shredded

1. Place rice and 310ml/11fl oz water in medium saucepan. Cover and bring to the boil. Reduce heat to low and simmer 14 minutes. Do not stir or lift lid. Remove from heat and let rice steam, covered, an additional 10 minutes.
2. Meanwhile, brown beef and garlic in a large nonstick frying pan over medium-high heat. Drain on kitchen paper to remove all fat.
3. Return meat mixture to pan and add mint, oregano, cumin and salt. Cook over medium heat 1 minute, stirring constantly.
4. Remove from heat. Stir in yogurt and cooked rice. Spoon onto centre of warm tortilla, top with shredded lettuce and roll up.

Note: To warm tortillas in the microwave, place flat in microwave and heat on medium 45–50 seconds until hot; do not overheat. Oven method: Wrap tortillas in aluminium foil and warm in 130°C/250°F/Gas mark ½ oven 10 minutes.

Tomato-Cucumber Salad

SERVES 4   total preparation time: **8 minutes**

4 medium tomatoes, sliced
4 medium cucumbers, thinly sliced
125ml/4fl oz fat-free salad dressing
4 large red or green lettuce leaves

1. Place tomatoes and cucumbers in a medium bowl and toss with salad dressing.
2. Place one lettuce leaf on each of four salad plates and top with equal portions of the tomato and cucumber mixture.

nutritional information per serving

	Calories	Protein	Carbs	Fat	Fibre	Sodium	Cholesterol	Calcium
Greek-Style Burrito								
	632	49 g	57 g	22 g	3 g	394 mg	73 mg	78 mg
Tomato-Cucumber Salad								
	93	4 g	20 g	0.5 g	5 g	22 mg	0 mg	74 mg
Steamed Green Beans								
	35	2 g	8 g	0 g	4 g	7 mg	0 mg	42 mg
Cantaloupe wedge								
	24	1g	6g	0 g	0.5g	6 mg	0 mg	8 mg
Meal Total								
	784	56 g	91 g	22.5 g (26%)	12.5 g	429 mg	73 mg	202 mg

Veal Chops with Papaya Salsa
White Rice
Parsley Carrot Coins (page 137)
Steamed Mangetouts
Steamed Green Beans
Melon chunks with sliced kiwi

Veal Chops with Papaya Salsa

SERVES 4   **total preparation time: 16 minutes**

Nonstick cooking spray
Four 170g/6oz boneless veal chops
1 large ripe papaya, peeled and chopped
227g can crushed pineapple (in juice or water)
1 teaspoon chopped fresh coriander
1 teaspoon lime juice

1. Spray a large nonstick frying pan with cooking spray. Sauté veal chops over medium-high heat 4 minutes on each side, or until cooked through.
2. Meanwhile, combine papaya, pineapple, coriander and lime juice in a large bowl. Mix well.
3. Place cooked chops on serving plates and top with papaya salsa.

White Rice

SERVES 4　　　　　　　　**total preparation time: 25 minutes**

140g/5oz uncooked white rice
¼ teaspoon salt

Place rice, salt and 310ml/11fl oz water in medium saucepan. Cover and bring to the boil. Reduce heat to low and simmer 14 minutes. Do not stir or lift lid. Remove from heat and let rice steam, covered, an additional 10 minutes.

Steamed Mangetouts

SERVES 4　　　　　　　　**total preparation time: 12 minutes**

450g/1lb mangetouts, trimmed

1. Fill a large saucepan with 5cm/2 inches water and bring to the boil.
2. Place mangetouts in steamer or colander and place in saucepan. Steam vegetables 5 minutes, or until crisp-tender.

Steamed Green Beans

SERVES 4   **total preparation time: 12 minutes**

450g/1lb green beans, trimmed

1. Fill a large saucepan with 5cm/2 inches water and bring to the boil.
2. Place beans in steamer or colander and place in saucepan. Steam 5 minutes, or until crisp-tender.

nutritional information per serving

	Calories	Protein	Carbs	Fat	Fibre	Sodium	Cholesterol	Calcium
Veal Chops with Papaya Salsa								
	410	53 g	13 g	14 g	2 g	133 mg	193 mg	79 mg
White Rice								
	105	2 g	23 g	0 g	0.5 g	0 mg	0 mg	3 mg
Parsley Carrot Coins								
	49	1 g	12 g	0 g	3 g	41 mg	0 mg	33 mg
Steamed Pea Pods								
	48	3 g	9 g	0 g	3 g	5 mg	0 mg	49 mg
Steamed Green Beans								
	35	2 g	8 g	0 g	4 g	7 mg	0 mg	42 mg
Melon chunks (85g/3oz) with sliced kiwi (½)								
	79	2 g	19 g	0.69 g	3 g	16 mg	0 mg	28 mg
Meal Total								
	717	63 g	84 g	15 g (19%)	15.5 g	202 mg	193 mg	234 mg

Menu

Mint-Glazed Lamb Chop
Baked Potato
Asparagus Spears
Fresh Cooked Beetroot
Tossed Salad (page 135)
Honeydew melon wedge

Mint-Glazed Lamb Chops

SERVES 4   **total preparation time: 25 minutes**

4 teaspoons cornflour
7g/¼oz fresh mint leaves, chopped
1½ tablespoons golden syrup
1 teaspoon grated lemon rind, yellow part only (with no white pith)
Four 200g/7oz lamb chops,1.5cm/¾ inch thick, trimmed of fat

1. Preheat grill.
2. In a small saucepan, combine 125ml/4fl oz water with the corn-flour. Add mint, syrup and grated lemon rind. Simmer over medium heat, stirring continually, 3–5 minutes, until thick and bubbly. Cook an additional 2 minutes. Remove from heat and set aside.
3. Place lamb chops on grill rack 3 inches from heat, and cook 4 minutes. Brush lightly with half the glaze. Turn, brush with remaining glaze and grill 4–5 minutes for medium.

Baked Potato

2 large floury baking potatoes, well scrubbed
4 tablespoons salsa

> *Oven method:* Preheat oven to 200°C/400°F/Gas mark 6. Prick each potato a few times with a fork. Place on a baking sheet and cook 50–60 minutes, or until soft when pricked with a fork. Cut in half and top each serving with 1 tablespoon salsa. *Microwave method:* Prick potatoes with a fork twice. Place side by side in centre of microwave oven. Cook on high 5–8 minutes, or until soft when pricked with a fork. Cut in half and top each serving with 1 tablespoon salsa.

Asparagus Spears

SERVES 4　　　　　　　total preparation time: **10 minutes**

680g/1½ lb asparagus

1. Fill a large saucepan with 5cm/2 inches water and bring to the boil.
2. Steam asparagus spears in colander over boiling water until crisp-tender, 6–8 minutes.

Fresh Cooked Beetroot

SERVES 4   total preparation time: **30 minutes**

680g/1½ lb fresh beetroot, with skins

1. Fill a large saucepan with enough to cover the beetroot and bring to the boil. Cook beetroot for 20 minutes or until tender when pierced with a fork. Drain and allow to cool.
2. When beetroot is cool enough to handle, peel and slice. Serve warm.

nutritional information per serving

	Calories	Protein	Carbs	Fat	Fibre	Sodium	Cholesterol	Calcium
Mint-Glazed Lamb Chop								
	393	47 g	14 g	15 g	0 g	151 mg	149 mg	35 mg
Baked Potato								
	104	2 g	24 g	0 g	2.5 g	49 mg	0 mg	17 mg
Asparagus Spears								
	39	4 g	8 g	0.5 g	3.5 g	3 mg	0 mg	36 mg
Fresh Cooked Beetroot								
	75	3 g	17 g	0 g	1 g	122 mg	0 mg	27 mg
Tossed Salad								
	88	5 g	18 g	1 g	5 g	35 mg	0 mg	73 mg
Honeydew melon wedge (⅛ melon)								
	56	1 g	15 g	0 g	1 g	16 mg	0 mg	10 mg
Meal Total								
	755	62 g	96 g	16.5 g (20%)	13 g	376 mg	149 mg	198 mg

Breakfasts

Most people find that Slim•Fast shakes and bars are best enjoyed for breakfast and lunch, with a sensible dinner to round off the day. But for those days when it's easiest to take along a shake for lunch and dinner – or for those days when you just would rather have a full plate of breakfast in front of you – here are three perfect options:

Menu
Blueberry Wholemeal Pancakes
dusted with 1 tablespoon icing sugar
Sliced fresh strawberries, 55g/2oz
Skimmed milk, 125ml/4fl oz

Blueberry Wholemeal Pancakes

SERVES 4   **total preparation time: 20 minutes**

115g/4oz plain flour
115g/4oz wholemeal flour
2 teaspoons baking powder
4 teaspoons granulated sugar
2 egg whites
400ml/14fl oz skimmed milk
1 tablespoon rapeseed oil
140g/5oz blueberries
Nonstick cooking spray

1. In a small bowl, combine plain flour, wholemeal flour, baking powder and sugar. Mix well and set aside.
2. In a large bowl, combine egg whites, milk and oil. Add flour mixture and stir until just moistened and lumpy. Gently fold in blueberries.
3. Spray a large nonstick frying pan with cooking spray and set over medium heat. For each pancake, spoon about 3 tablespoons batter into the hot pan, making a small circle. Cook until pancakes are bubbly on top, 4 minutes. Flip and cook until browned on bottom, 2–3 additional minutes.

nutritional information per serving

	Calories	Protein	Carbs	Fat	Fibre	Sodium	Cholesterol	Calcium
Blueberry Whole Wheat Pancakes								
	275	11 g	49.5 g	4 g	4 g	330 mg	2 mg	281 mg
Icing sugar								
	24	0 g	6 g	0 g	0 g	0 mg	0 mg	0 mg
Strawberries								
	25	0.5 g	6 g	0.5 g	2 g	1 mg	0 mg	12 mg
Skimmed milk (125ml/4fl oz)								
	42	4 g	5.5 g	0.1 g	0 g	58 mg	2 mg	139 mg
Meal Total								
	366	15.5 g	67.0 g	4.6 g (11%)	6 g	389 mg	4 mg	432 mg

Apple Oat Bran Muffins

Fresh orange juice, 125ml/4fl oz

Cantaloupe wedge, ⅛ melon

Low-fat cottage cheese with pineapple, 115g/4oz

Apple Oat Bran Muffins

MAKES 10   total preparation time: **30 minutes**

1 medium tart apple, peeled, cored and thinly sliced

1 tablespoon lemon juice

170g/6oz plain flour

55g/2oz oat bran

1 tablespoon baking powder

1½ teaspoons ground cinnamon

¼ teaspoon ground nutmeg

250g/9oz unsweetened prepared apple sauce

125ml/4fl oz skimmed milk

55g/2oz firmly packed brown sugar

1 egg white

70g/2½oz raisins

1. Preheat oven to 220°C/425°F/Gas mark 7. Line a ten-hole muffin tray with paper cases.
2. In a small bowl, toss apple slices with lemon juice and set aside. In a large bowl, combine flour, oat bran, baking powder, cinnamon and nutmeg. In a separate bowl, mix apple sauce, milk, sugar, egg white, raisins and the apple slices with lemon juice. Combine the wet and dry ingredients and mix well.
3. Spoon the batter into muffin cups and bake 15–20 minutes, or until a toothpick inserted in centre of muffins comes out clean.

nutritional information per serving

	Calories	Protein	Carbs	Fat	Fibre	Sodium	Cholesterol	Calcium
Apple Oat Bran Muffin								
	133	4 g	32 g	1 g	3 g	161 mg	0 mg	112 mg
Orange juice								
	51	1 g	12 g	0 g	0 g	1 mg	0 mg	12 mg
Cantaloupe wedge								
	24	1 g	6 g	0 g	0.5 g	6 mg	0 mg	8 mg
Cottage cheese								
	110	11 g	11 g	1.5 g	0 g	291 mg	10 mg	40 mg
Meal Total								
	318	17 g	61 g	2.5 g (7%)	3.5 g	459 mg	10 mg	172 mg

Menu

Spicy Turkey Breakfast Patties
Honeydew wedge, ⅛ melon
Wholemeal toast, 1 slice
Reduced-calorie fruit spread, 1 tablespoon

Spicy Turkey Breakfast Patties

SERVES 4   total preparation time: **15 minutes**

½ small onion, finely diced
450g/1lb minced turkey breast meat
1 teaspoon chopped fresh rosemary or ½ teaspoon dried
2 teaspoons chopped fresh sage or 1 teaspoon dried
½ teaspoon black pepper

1. Place onion in small bowl and cover with clingfilm. Microwave on high (100 per cent power) 45 seconds. In a large bowl, combine turkey, rosemary, sage and pepper. Add onions and mix well. Form into 8 patties, each 7cm/3 inches in diameter and 5mm/¼ inch thick.
2. Place patties in large nonstick frying pan and cook over high heat 1 minute; turn and cook 1 more minute. Reduce heat to low and cook, turning occasionally, until golden brown and cooked through, 3 more minutes.

nutritional information per serving

	Calories	Protein	Carbs	Fat	Fibre	Sodium	Cholesterol	Calcium
Spicy Turkey Breakfast Patties								
	176	20 g	1.5 g	9 g	0.5 g	107 mg	90 mg	23 mg
Honeydew wedge								
	56	1 g	15 g	0 g	1 g	16 mg	0 mg	10 mg
Wholemeal toast								
	69	3 g	13 g	1 g	2 g	148 mg	0 mg	20 mg
Reduced-calorie fruit spread								
	20	0 g	5 g	0 g	0 g	20 mg	0 mg	0 mg
Meal Total								
	321	24 g	34.5 g	10 g (19%)	3.5 g	291 mg	90 mg	53 mg

Speciality Shakes and Smoothies

One of the great things about Slim•Fast shakes is that you can dress them up in so many different ways. This selection of recipes represents only a few of the delicious health drinks that can be made quickly and easily with Ultra Slim•Fast shakes and powders. Don't feel limited to this list – it's just a start! Get creative; invent your own sensational shakes and smoothies based on your favourite ingredients and flavour combinations. Experiment and share your great-tasting recipes with a friend. The healthy possibilities are endless!

Cappuccino Smoothie

1 heaped scoop Chocolate Royale Slim•Fast powder
250ml/8fl oz skimmed milk, chilled
1 teaspoon instant coffee
6 ice cubes

Blend all ingredients together in a liquidizer or food processor for 40 seconds. Pour into a tall glass and enjoy.

Chocolate Mint Shake

1 heaped scoop Chocolate Royale Slim•Fast powder
250ml/8fl oz skimmed milk, chilled
¼ teaspoon peppermint extract
4 ice cubes

Blend all ingredients together in a liquidizer or food processor for 40 seconds. Pour into a tall glass and enjoy.

Quick Fudge Pops

1 heaped scoop Chocolate Royale Slim•Fast powder
250ml/8fl oz skimmed milk, chilled
1 teaspoon cocoa powder
Artificial sweetener to taste
4 ice cubes

1. Blend all ingredients together in a liquidizer or food processor for 40 seconds. Pour into ice-lolly moulds. Place in freezer.
2. When pops are half-frozen (about 15 minutes) insert sticks. Allow to freeze completely.
3. To unfreeze, run warm water on the outside of the mould. Enjoy!

Milk Chocolate Freeze

1 heaped scoop Chocolate Royale Slim•Fast powder
2 teaspoons cocoa powder
200ml/7fl oz skimmed milk, chilled
Artificial sweetener to taste
¼ teaspoon vanilla essence
10 ice cubes

1. Combine all ingredients in a liquidizer or food processor and blend for 40 seconds. Transfer to a metal mixing bowl and place in freezer for about 2 hours.
2. Remove frozen mixture from freezer and allow to sit 10 minutes. Transfer contents back to the liquidizer or food processor and blend until smooth. Serve immediately.

Double Strawberry Cooler

1 heaped scoop Strawberry Supreme Slim•Fast powder
250ml/8fl oz skimmed milk, chilled
70g/2½ oz fresh or frozen strawberries
6 ice cubes

Blend all ingredients together in a liquidizer or food processor for 40 seconds. Pour into a tall glass and enjoy.

Strawberry Banana Sipper

1 heaped scoop Strawberry Supreme Slim•Fast powder
250ml/8fl oz skimmed milk, chilled
½ banana, peeled and cut into slices
4 ice cubes

Blend all ingredients together in a liquidizer or food processor for 40 seconds. Pour into a tall glass and enjoy.

Orange Creamsicle

1 heaped scoop French Vanilla Slim•Fast powder
125ml/4fl oz fresh orange juice, chilled
125ml/4fl oz skimmed milk, chilled
115g/4oz very low fat natural yogurt
4 ice cubes

Blend all ingredients together in a liquidizer or food processor for 40 seconds. Pour into a tall glass and enjoy.

Vanilla Tapioca Pudding

1 tablespoon instant tapioca
250ml/8fl oz skimmed milk
1 heaped scoop French Vanilla Slim•Fast powder
½ teaspoon vanilla essence
A pinch of ground nutmeg

1. Combine tapioca and milk in saucepan. Allow to sit 5 minutes. Cook mixture over medium heat, stirring frequently until mixture reaches a full boil.
2. Remove from heat, transfer to a liquidizer or food processor and add the Slim•Fast and vanilla essence. Blend 30 seconds on medium speed.
3. Let cool at room temperature for 20 minutes for warm tapioca, or refrigerate until cool for chilled tapioca. Sprinkle with nutmeg before serving.

Sunrise Shake

1 can Slim•Fast French Vanilla Ready-to-Drink Shake, chilled
45g/1½ oz fresh peach, cut into chunks
45g/1½ oz fresh strawberries, halved
6 ice cubes

Blend all ingredients together in a liquidizer or food processor for 40 seconds. Pour into a tall glass and enjoy.

Chocolate-Dipped Strawberry Shake

1 can Ultra Slim•Fast Rich Chocolate Royale Ready-to-Drink Shake,
    chilled
70g/2½ oz frozen strawberries
6 ice cubes

Blend all ingredients together in a liquidizer or food processor for
40 seconds. Pour into a tall glass and enjoy.

Cherry Vanilla Shake

1 can Slim•Fast French Vanilla Ready-to-Drink Shake, chilled
85g/3oz canned or frozen black cherries (be sure to select the no-
    sugar variety)
1 teaspoon vanilla essence
6 ice cubes

Blend all ingredients together in a liquidizer or food processor for
40 seconds. Pour into a tall glass and enjoy.

7

your exercise
and relaxation makeover

Now that you've read all about the eating plan, you may be tempted to focus just on changing your eating habits and skipping the rest of the Slim•Fast Makeover. After all, if you've dieted before, that's probably all you did – put different kinds or smaller amounts of food into your mouth. But you know how successful that was, right?

So now it's time to do things differently. It's time to make changes that will actually enrich your life – enabling you to have a healthier, more adventurous and more enjoyable life. And that's what the makeover is all about: putting both your body and your mind on the right track. Of course, it's possible to lose weight simply by eating better for a limited period of time; but if you want to keep the weight off for good – and look and feel as good as you should – you've got to change your mind-set and lifestyle as well.

After giving yourself the makeover, you'll no longer feel compelled to park in the closest parking space, or take the lift at work rather than the stairs. You'll be less tempted to use food to ease your boredom or help you cope with a stressful day. You'll find that you're less obsessive about food as you turn to other ways to relax and get enjoyment out of life.

This chapter will help you create your own exercise plan and develop your own relaxation plan. These are the very components that are usually missing from diet plans, but they're essential for upping the odds of success. They work hand in hand to combat food cravings and improve your overall well-being. For instance, combining exercise and relaxation can ease the PMS food cravings and mood swings, and help you through a stressful period at work – two things that can sabotage even the best-laid weight-loss plans. In terms of your body chemistry, both exercise and relaxation lower your body's level of stress hormones and boost your level of chemicals such as endorphins and serotonin, which can make you feel happy and calm. Both are also great for your health and may help lower your risk of heart disease and other illnesses.

Countless Slim•Fast users have found that exercise is a key component in weight loss. They've also found that exercise and weight loss build on each other: losing weight improves your ability to exercise and enables you to do activities you may never have thought you could manage.

After you've read through the exercises on the following pages, it's your turn to use them as the building blocks of your own exercise programme. Note in your personal makeover diary every new exercise you try, as this will help you learn more about what kind of workout will work best for you.

Creating Your Personal Exercise Plan

Exercise, of course, is key to successful weight loss; combined with a balanced diet, it can help you take off weight and create a more toned and efficient body. And yet many people have spent years shying away from physical activity. Beginning an exercise programme can be daunting – especially if you don't know enough about what to do.

This plan is designed to teach you the basics. You will learn three different types of exercises – aerobic activity, resistance training and stretching – all of which your body needs. You'll become stronger, feel more energetic, and develop a firmer, fitter body. Exercise can be just as easy as changing your eating habits. What's more, once you see how good it makes you feel, you'll find you can't live without it.

If you're already following a workout programme, feel free to continue the exercises that are working for you – but you can also use this as an opportunity to try something new. Buy yourself a new workout video, or take the spinning class that's on offer at the gym. You may learn something from the advice in the following pages – maybe you're not stretching as much as you should, or you're neglecting to strengthen your muscles through resistance training.

This plan will show you that exercise doesn't need to make you grunt and groan to be beneficial. Contrary to the 'no-pain-no-gain' philosophy many people espouse, it has been shown that moderate amounts of activity *can* provide health benefits and weight loss to people who previously were sedentary.

On this plan you'll have a simple goal: get one hour of exercise per day. As we've discussed, this isn't as difficult as it sounds – especially if you accumulate activity throughout the day. Walk fifteen minutes each way to take your child to school every morning and you'll only need thirty minutes on the exercise bike in the evening.

If you've never exercised before and you are severely overweight, it'll probably take you several weeks before you can handle sixty minutes of activity each day. That's okay. Work your way up slowly. Start with a fifteen-minute walk on the first day and gradually increase the time as your stamina increases. What's important to realize is that any amount of exercise is beneficial. More exercise is better than some, and some is better than none.

Don't think of exercise as a formal regime you're forcing yourself to follow until you lose the weight and you can give it up. Like the

Slim•Fast eating plan, the exercise plan is a life change that you'll want to stay with because it makes you feel good. You just need to allow yourself a few weeks to get into the exercise groove. If you have to skip a workout one day, don't beat yourself up about it. Just find ways to add little bursts of activity into your days, like taking the stairs at work instead of the lift. The important thing is to stay committed.

Making Exercise – and Love – a Part of Your Life

For me, exercise is always very tough to start, especially with my schedule constantly changing. When I first started trying to work a serious exercise regime into my life, I had to start all over again time after time; I'd get going with a new gym regime, then work would take me off somewhere else, and I'd get thrown off my rhythm. The big problem was, every time I stopped I felt I was reverting to ground zero; it was as if everything I'd done so far was for nothing, and I'd feel that old familiar depression creeping in, slow but steady.

Now I realize that the problem wasn't with me – it was with the inflexible, unrealistic demands I was trying to impose on my life. That's why the Slim•Fast programme puts so much emphasis on creating a personal programme that works for you. Whether it's going to the gym, doing aerobics at home, or simply taking a good hard walk through your neighbourhood every day, what's most important isn't what kind of exercise you do – it's that you get it done.

Now I'm as faithful to my goals as I can be, but I don't chastise myself if I miss a day. And what always draws me back to my personal exercise plan is remembering how good I feel about my *self* – about my self-image – when I'm exercising regularly. And when I come back to it, after a couple of days it's like magic – I breathe better, think better, sleep better, and have infinitely more energy. Above all, I like myself better, and maybe for good reason – because, for all of the above reasons, I'm a kinder and better person when I'm taking care of myself.

And don't forget about sex! I don't know if you're the same way, but when I'm not getting enough exercise, the last thing I'm interested in is the idea of sharing my unclothed, unfit body with my lover. Yikes! But after a few days of exercise, all those negative feelings disappear. Suddenly I'm full of optimism, peace of mind, and positive energy. And *voilà!* When you feel that way, your whole life is enhanced. And suddenly you have so much energy you feel like sharing it with others; next thing you know, you're interested, you're caring – and you're *sexy*. You twinkle for them. And you start sharing your joy ... the sexiest feeling of all.

Step 1: Get Your Calorie Burn

Steady or aerobic exercise – like walking, cycling, running and swimming – makes your body burn calories quickly, helping you shed excess pounds. It also strengthens your heart and helps build muscle. You'll probably also notice that you feel energized and invigorated after a workout – a boost researchers attribute to increases in the brain's level of endorphins.

It's time to choose an aerobic activity that you'll be comfortable doing on a regular basis, four or five days a week. If you haven't exercised before, you should choose a simple activity like walking or riding on a stationary bike. Once you've improved your fitness level, you can move on to more challenging things such as aerobics classes or tennis lessons. Unless you're in good physical shape, be aware that your first few weeks of exercise will be tough. You'll probably be huffing and puffing after just a few minutes of exertion, and you may not be having much fun as you try to get your body to do things it isn't used to.

As you build your endurance, though, you'll be amazed as your body's capabilities grow before your eyes. Where you could once barely manage a ten-minute walk, you'll find within weeks that a thirty-minute walk becomes a piece of cake.

Here are a few suggestions you can use as a guide for choosing an aerobic activity. After a brief description of each activity, you'll find recommended stretches you should do before and after your workouts. Instructions and illustrations for these stretches are found in the stretching section in Step 2. You'll also find the calculated calorie burn that you'll get from doing an hour of each activity. The calculation is based on a 67 kilogram (150 pound) person; if you weigh more you'll burn more calories, if you weigh less you'll burn less. Remember: your goal is to get about an hour of activity each day, to burn an estimated 250–300 calories.

Aerobics

Aerobics is a combination of dance and calisthenics, and includes such variations as step aerobics, slide aerobics, and movement classes influenced by everything from jazz to hip-hop to funk.

Benefits to your body Aerobics helps tone muscles throughout your entire body while burning calories at the same time, so it's also great for weight loss.

It's easy You can learn techniques from the class or video instructor, so you don't need to be physically fit to begin (although you need to choose a level of activity that's within your capabilities). As you become fitter, you can progress to a more advanced class or video, so you don't get bored if the workouts get too easy.

Format Most aerobics classes and videos include a short warm-up and stretching period, a thirty-minute workout, stretching and cool-down, and a short muscle-toning session.

What you'll need Trainers with ankle support designed specifically for aerobics, or cross-trainers. Wear exercise clothes made from a synthetic material (not cotton), which will help keep sweat away from your skin. A sports bra is essential for women.

Warm-up and stretches Most aerobics classes and videos include a warm-up and stretches at the beginning of the workout. If they don't, march on the spot for about five to ten minutes before stretching. Be sure to stretch the following muscle groups after your warm-up to reduce your risk of injury and after your cool-down to reduce soreness and increase flexibility:

Quadriceps: large muscles in front of thighs
Hamstrings: large muscles in back of thighs
Gluteus: buttock muscles
Calves
Triceps: muscles in back of upper arms
Biceps: muscles in front of the arms

Cool-down If your instructor fails to do one, walk around for five to ten minutes to allow your heart rate to descend gradually.

Calorie burn 340 calories per hour, moderate intensity (based on a 67kg/150lb person).

Walking

Walking is one of the safest and healthiest exercises you can do. A recent study from Harvard University found that walking briskly for three hours a week can cut the risk of heart disease in women by as much as 40 per cent – equivalent to the benefits of regular aerobics, jogging, or other vigorous physical activity. Walking is also the cheapest, easiest form of exercise. All you have to do is open your door and get moving!

Benefits to your body Walking strengthens the hips, thighs, buttocks and legs. The faster your pace, the more calories you burn. The longer you walk, the more you build up your endurance. Besides reducing your risk of heart disease, walking may lower high blood pressure. And walking two or more miles a day can help older people live longer, according to a recent study. Walking also helps prevent osteoporosis, since it's a weight-bearing activity. Of course, it's also a great way to lose weight!

It's convenient You can do it just about anywhere, at home on the treadmill or outdoors to get you to and from work. Whether you're alone or with friends, you can adjust your pace for almost any fitness level. To get a good workout, though, walk as briskly as you can. You should be breathing hard and sweating without feeling discomfort. Since it's easy on the joints, you can walk even if injury keeps you from more strenuous activity.

Warm-up and stretches Go at about half speed for the first five minutes of your walk to allow your muscles to warm up. Be sure to stretch the following muscle groups after your warm-up to reduce your risk of injury and after your cool-down to reduce soreness and increase flexibility:

Quadriceps
Gluteus
Hamstrings
Calves

Cool-down Slow your pace at the end of the walk to allow your heart rate to descend gradually.

Calorie burn 272 calories per hour, brisk pace of 3.5 mph (based on 67kg/150lb person).

Cycling

Getting out and cycling is one of the fastest ways to get physically fit. Even if you haven't cycled in years, the cliché holds true – you never forget how.

Benefits to your body Cycling works your leg muscles, buttocks and calves. And a recent study found that cycling for just thirty minutes six times a month may reduce the risk of premature death by more than half. Cycling is also gentle on the body and ideal for people who have joint or back problems.

It's a mode of transportation You can cycle into town or to work, so it's easy to fit in workouts. You can also go for day-long outings with friends or family, either on quiet roads or off-road. To stay in shape in between jaunts, take a spinning class at the gym or ride a stationary bike at home.

What you need A road bike, mountain bike, or hybrid bike. A road bike has thinner tyres and a lighter frame, so it's easier to achieve speed. A mountain bike is heavier, lets you sit upright, and is less vulnerable to flat tires. Hybrid bikes let you sit upright and have sturdier wheels, but like road bikes, they're lighter. They're a good compromise for beginners. You also need a helmet to protect yourself from serious head injuries. Wear comfortable clothes and trainers.

Warm-up and stretches Pedal at a comfortable pace for five to ten minutes until you break into a light sweat. This will warm up your muscles. Be sure to stretch the following muscle groups after your warm-up to reduce your risk of injury and after your cool-down to reduce soreness and increase flexibility:

Calves

Gluteus

Hamstrings

Quadriceps

Upper and lower back

Cool-down During the last few minutes of your ride, slow your pace to half-speed to let your heart rate descend gradually.

Calorie burn 408 calories per hour, moderate intensity (based on 67kg/150lb person).

Swimming

Swimming is one of the few fitness activities that gives you a great workout without jarring your body. It's great for people of all fitness levels – especially beginners.

Benefits to your body Along with strengthening your heart, it works your legs, arms, buttocks and abdominal muscles. It's great for building stamina and muscle tone without overtaxing your joints.

What you need A snug-fitting suit designed for athletic swimming, goggles to keep the chlorine out of your eyes and a swimming cap if your hair is long.

Warm-up and stretches Get moving for five or ten minutes before you begin your workout. March on the spot, walk to the pool, or start out with slow, easy strokes. Be sure to stretch the following muscle groups after your warm-up to reduce your risk of injury and after your cool-down to reduce soreness and increase flexibility:

Quadriceps

Gluteus

Hamstrings

Calves

Triceps

Shoulders

Cool-down When you're done, have a leisurely swim for a few minutes before getting out of the pool to give your muscles a chance to cool down.

Calorie burn 544 calories per hour (based on 67kg/150lb person).

Tennis

Tennis makes even a hard workout feel like fun. Having a partner to compete with keeps you challenged, while your legs get a workout from the constant back-and-forth movement.

Benefits to your body Tennis makes your joints more flexible, particularly in the hips and the shoulder used to serve. It also develops and tones your muscles, especially the quadriceps, hamstrings, calves, arms, shoulders and upper back. As a bonus, you'll experience an improvement in hand-eye coordination, balance and agility – and, of course, you'll get a cardiovascular workout.

It's a social event Tennis is a great way to socialize. You can play with up to three other people at a time or sign up for mini tournaments. And the increasing number of indoor courts means you shouldn't have to forego a game because of the weather.

What you need If you've never played tennis before, you should go to a certified teaching professional to learn the proper techniques for hitting the ball, so that you avoid injury. They can recommend the right racket for your playing style and skill level. Aerobic activities, strength training and stretching will get you in the necessary condition for tennis.

Warm-up and stretches You should warm up your muscles for five to ten minutes before playing to lower your risk of injury. Gently lob the ball back and forth a few times. Be sure to stretch the following muscle groups after your warm-up to reduce your risk of injury and after your cool-down to reduce soreness and increase flexibility:

Calves
Forearms
Gluteus
Hamstrings
Obliques
Quadriceps
Shoulders
Triceps
Upper and lower back

Cool-down If you've played a light game, walk around the court to collect stray balls. If you've played intensely enough to get you sweating and breathing heavily, walk around until your heart rate returns to normal.

Calorie burn 340 calories per hour (based on 67kg/150lb person).

Spinning

Spinning, also called studio or indoor cycling, is offered as a group class in many gyms and is extremely challenging. With its loud music, dim lights, instructors shouting out orders and the sound of many bikes working together, spinning has taken the fitness world by storm.

Benefits to your body Spinning is an excellent way to lose weight because it burns a huge amount of calories. It tones your quadriceps, hamstrings, calves, hips and abdominals. It also improves your cardiovascular fitness and endurance. During your first few weeks, though, you should take a spinning class for beginners; it's easy to overexert yourself trying to keep up with a pack of advanced spinners.

It's low-impact and easier on the joints Compared to other high-intensity exercises like running and aerobics, spinning is low-impact and less likely to cause muscle injuries or joint problems. You may also find the team aspect appealing and fun. You should, however, be in moderately good physical shape. Any aerobic exercise like cycling on your own time or walking can help you get in shape for a class.

What you need Wear workout clothes made from a synthetic material to help keep sweat away from your skin. Get a comfortable pair of cycle shorts with padding in the seat area, which provides some needed cushioning. Have a towel on hand to mop up sweat from your face and hands.

Warm-up and stretches Most instructors start with a warm-up, but if they don't, try a five-minute warm-up on a stationary bike before class yourself or take a brisk walk or jog. Be sure to stretch the following muscle groups after your warm-up to reduce your risk of injury and after your cool-down to reduce soreness and increase flexibility:

Quadriceps
Gluteus
Hamstrings
Calves

Cool-down Allow your heart rate to descend gradually by walking around the studio or continuing to ride the stationary bike at a slow to moderately slow pace.

Calorie burn 476 calories per hour (based on a 67kg/150lb person).

Hiking

Hiking is a great workout for all fitness levels if you enjoy the out-doors. Beginners can go on flat walks, while the experienced can head off for more mountainous terrain. If you're a complete beginner, joining a local ramblers or walkers group is a good way to get started.

Benefits to your body As long as you keep up a steady pace, you can burn off a lot of calories and fat through hiking. Hiking will build your endurance and will help build muscle strength, particularly in the quadriceps, hamstrings, gluteus muscles and calves. It will also strengthen your bones. Carrying a rucksack will help you burn even more.

It allows time for reflection Taking in the awe-inspiring beauty of nature will invigorate you and allow your mind to escape the stresses of daily life. Hiking also enables you to challenge your mind by plotting your own course and keeping yourself from getting lost. Hiking is a great group activity, though you may also enjoy it alone. If you're a solo hiker, be sure to tell someone where you're going and when you intend to get back in case you get lost or injured.

What you need You'll need to invest in a pair of proper hiking boots. Ankle support is important – as is cushioning in the arch and heel, since the terrain can be rocky and uneven. Try on boots with the same socks you're planning to wear when you hike. Break in your new hiking boots at least a week before your trip. You also need waterproofs, a water bottle, and an emergency kit in case you get lost (with extra food like a nutrition bar, water, a flashlight, a compass, a first-aid kit, and matches or a lighter).

Warm-up and stretches Be sure to stretch the following muscle groups after your warm-up to reduce your risk of injury and after your cool-down to reduce soreness and increase flexibility:

Quadriceps
Gluteus
Hamstrings
Calves

Cool-down Before you end your hike, slow down to a stroll for four or five minutes to allow your heart rate to descend gradually.

Calorie burn 408 calories per hour (based on 67kg/150lb person).

Step 2: Stretch It to the Max

When you think about exercise, you probably don't think about stretching. Many exercisers neglect to stretch before and after workouts, writing it off as a waste of time. The truth is, although stretching itself doesn't directly contribute to weight loss, it has a host of other benefits. Stretching can enhance your performance during workouts by increasing your range of motion and improving your coordination; it can also help you avoid injuries that can sideline you for weeks.

Stretching for five to ten minutes before and after workouts can help avoid some of the ravages of ageing – from decreased flexibility and poor balance to stiff joints. Regular stretching will relieve muscle tension, improve circulation and enhance muscle tone. What's more, it makes you feel great!

A complete stretching routine appears below. It's best to warm up for three to five minutes before stretching to avoid pulling a muscle. Do any continuous movement that gets your heart rate elevated, like walking up and down the stairs a few times or jogging in place. *When you stretch, focus on the muscle being stretched and hold each stretch for ten to fifteen seconds.* Repeat each stretch three to five times. Try not to bounce, since this can force the joints past their natural range of motion, causing sprains of the ligaments or tendons. Stretch to a point where you feel a mild tension.

Chest

Sit or stand with your hands clasped behind your back. With your hands intertwined, raise your hands upward a few inches until you feel mild tension between your shoulder blades and in your upper chest.

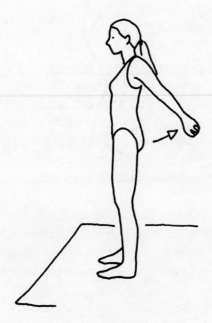

Upper Back

Stand with your arms extended in front of you at shoulder height.
Hold your hands together, fingers intertwined, with palms facing out.
Round your shoulders and reach away from your chest. Keep your
knees slightly bent throughout the stretch. You should feel the stretch
across your entire upper back.

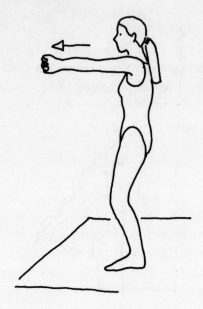

Calves

Stand with your hands and feet against a wall and take a large step back with one leg. Keep your legs aligned with your hips. With your front leg bent and your back leg straight, press the heel of your back leg into the floor. Press your hands into the wall for support, feeling the stretch in the back of your calf. Repeat on the other leg.

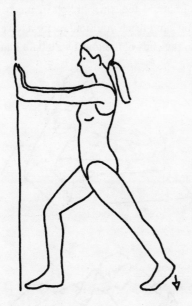

Hamstrings

Sit with your legs straight in front of you, with your feet relaxed (don't flex or point them). Bend one leg so that the bottom of your foot touches the inner thigh of the straight leg. Keeping your back straight and your chest out, bring your forehead toward the shin of the straight leg. Reach for your foot with both hands. Repeat on the other leg. You should feel this stretch in the back of your thigh. Variation: If you can't reach your foot, place a towel around your foot and hold on to the ends of the towel with both hands.

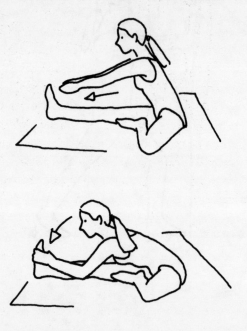

Triceps

Sit or stand and extend both arms overhead. Bend one arm behind your head and gently push down on the elbow with the opposite hand. Repeat on the opposite arm. You should feel the stretch on the back of your upper arm.

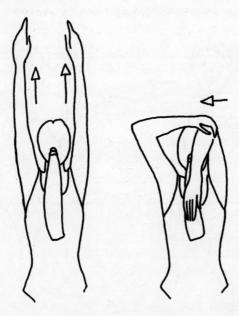

Shoulders

Place your right arm across your chest, keeping your arm straight and your shoulders down. Bring your left arm up from underneath, and place your left hand just above the right elbow. Pull your right arm gently toward your body. Repeat on the other side. You should feel the stretch across the top of your shoulder and upper arm.

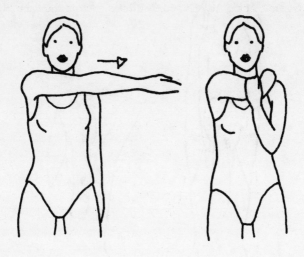

Quadriceps

Standing on your right leg with your left leg lifted behind you, grab the ankle of your left leg with your left hand and pull your heel up behind you toward your buttock. Keep your knees close together and your back straight (not arched). Repeat on the other side. If you have sore knees, loop a towel around your ankle and keep your knee bent at a 90-degree angle. You should feel this stretch in the front of the thigh.

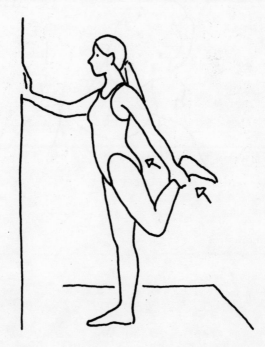

Neck

Slowly drop your ear toward your right shoulder. When you reach a comfortable tension, gently lower your left shoulder. You should feel the stretch on the left side of your neck. Repeat the stretch on the other side. Now drop your chin toward your chest and hold. Keep your shoulders back. You should feel this stretch down the back of your neck and in your upper back.

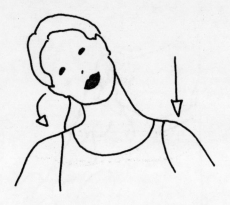

Lower Back

Lie on your back with your knees bent and your feet flat on the floor. Keeping your knees bent, reach behind both legs under your thighs and bring your thighs into your chest, lifting your feet off the floor. Your lower back should remain on the floor. Your legs should feel relaxed through the entire move. You should feel this stretch in your lower back and buttocks.

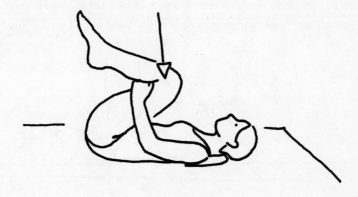

Gluteus (Buttocks)

Lie on your back with both knees bent and your feet flat on the floor. Take your right foot in your left hand (wrapping your hand under your foot so that your fingertips are on its outside edge) and hold your leg (with your knee bent) in the air about one to three feet above your chest. Exhale and slowly pull your foot over to the side and up toward your head. You should feel the stretch in your buttocks. Repeat on the other side. If you have sore knees, wrap a towel around your ankle and use the ends of the towel to pull your leg up.

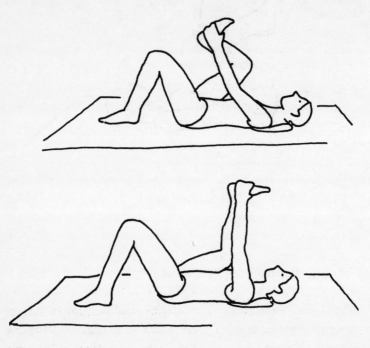

Convenient Calorie Burners

Having trouble fitting a full hour of exercise into your daily routine? Here's a chart that highlights some simple and convenient exercises and activities that may be easier to fit into a busy day. Next to each activity is the calculated calorie burn (remember, you want to burn about 300 calories per day).

Activity	Calories Burned (for 67kg/150lb person)
Brisk 15 minute walk	68
Sit-ups and push-ups for 10 minutes	91
Walking upstairs for 10 minutes	91
Dancing for 20 minutes	93
Cleaning your house for 30 minutes (vacuuming, mopping, dusting, cleaning bathrooms)	119
Light outdoor play with kids for 15 minutes	68
Lawn mowing for 40 minutes	250
Gardening for 20 minutes	113
Running on the spot for 10 minutes	91
Skipping with a rope slowly for 15 minutes	136

Step 3: Pump Yourself Up

You've probably heard about the benefits of building muscle through strength or resistance training (the terms are synonymous). Resistance training makes you stronger and can make day-to-day tasks like carrying groceries much easier. It'll also make aerobic workouts much easier, as your muscles propel your body from place to place.

What you may not know is that strength training actually helps you burn more calories throughout the day, because muscle requires more calories to maintain than fat. Boosting your metabolism this way will help you lose weight and maintain the loss. In the long term, strength training can help prevent bone loss and protect against osteoporosis; it can also offset the increases in weight that usually occur with age as your metabolism starts to decline.

You may have avoided strength training in the past out of fear of developing bulging muscles. But there isn't a very big risk of developing large muscles if you're doing the right amount of weight-lifting. What you should see is greater muscle definition and a sculpted look as your body gains tone. Unfortunately, though, you can't spot-reduce your stomach through abdominal crunches or your butt and thighs through squats. Aerobic activity will help burn off fat in all the areas of your body, while resistance training will give you a more defined look.

If you don't have access to a gym's wide range of exercise machines, you'll need to get some basic equipment to get a full strength training workout. If you're just getting started, you can purchase a set of exercise (resistance) bands in a sports equipment shop. For weights, you can start by holding heavy soup cans or filled litre-size water bottles. Once these weights get too light, you should purchase a starter set of dumbbells. You can buy a new set reasonably cheaply, or try the local classifieds for a second-hand set.

The following exercises work all your major muscle groups. Aim to do this workout two to three times a week – though not on consecutive days, since muscles need a day to recover in between workouts.

One note: You may find that your rate of weight loss slows down as you begin to resistance-train. If you've been following your eating plan carefully, you're probably building muscle and lowering your percentage of body fat – which is, of course, a good thing. For reassurance, you can monitor your efforts by getting your body fat percentage tested – most health clubs offer these tests – but you should also be able to tell simply by monitoring your waistline and how well your clothes fit.

Lunge

Works gluteus muscles, quadriceps and hamstrings.

Stand with your feet together and your hands at your sides. Take an exaggerated step backward with your right leg.

Bend your right knee slowly, lowering your body close to the floor. Keep your right knee directly over your right foot and your back straight. Most of your weight will be over your right foot. You should feel the strain in your hips and thighs, not your knees, ankles, or back.

Hold position for one second and slowly return to starting position. Perform eight to twelve repetitions. Then do a set on your left leg.

Variation: Once you can do twelve repetitions with good form, you can make the exercise harder by holding a dumbbell in each hand.

Weight room equivalent: Leg press

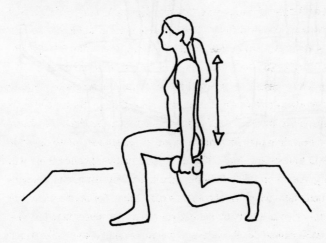

Knee Extension

Works your quadriceps.

Sit on a chair with your knees bent. Attach an exercise band to your right ankle and the rear leg of the chair. The band should be taut but not stretched.

Slowly lift your right foot, straightening your leg until it's parallel to the floor. Hold for one second.

Lower your foot back to the starting position. Do eight to twelve repetitions, then switch legs and repeat on the left leg.

Variation: Use ankle weights instead of exercise bands.
Weight room equivalent: Leg extension

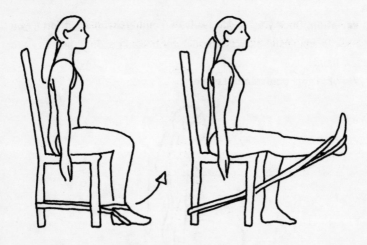

Leg Curl

Strengthens your hamstrings.

Stand near a wall or a table. Attach one end of a resistance band to your right ankle and step on the other end with your left foot. To maintain your balance, place your feet no more than shoulder-width apart.

Keeping your knee still, bend your right leg and pull your foot as close to your buttocks as you can. Use the wall or table for support if necessary. Hold for one second, then slowly lower your foot to the ground.

Perform eight to twelve repetitions. Switch feet and do a set with your left leg.

Variation: Use ankle weights instead of exercise bands.
Weight room equivalent: Seated or prone leg curl

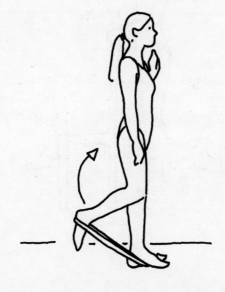

Toe Raise

Works your calves.

Rest your hands on the back of a chair and position your feet straight in front of you about shoulder-width apart. Your toes should be facing forward or slightly outward.

Slowly raise your heels so that you're standing on the balls of your feet. Hold for one second. Slowly lower your heels to the ground. Do eight to twelve repetitions.

Weight room equivalent: Seated calf

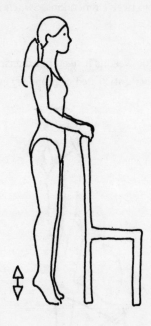

Push-up

Works your chest muscles, as well as shoulders and triceps.

Lie face down on the floor with your hands flat on the floor, almost underneath your shoulders but a little wider apart.

Push your body off the floor, using your toes as a pivot point. Keep your back straight and your head in line with your body. (Beginners can do modified push-ups: use your knees as the pivot point. Keep your toes on the floor or bend your knees at a 90-degree angle and cross your ankles.)

When your elbows are fully straightened, hold for one second. Slowly lower yourself to within one inch of the floor. You should feel the effort in your chest, shoulders and triceps, not your neck. Without letting your chest touch the floor, do another push-up. Do eight to twelve repetitions.

Weight room equivalent: Bench press

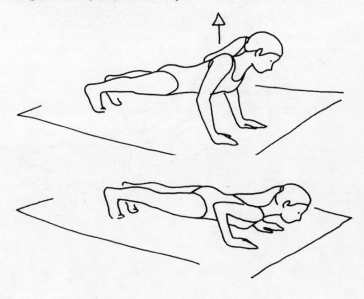

Seated Row

Targets the upper back muscles.

Loop a resistance band around your feet. Sit on the floor with your legs straight in front of you. Grasp the ends of the band in your hands. It should have only slight tension.

Slowly pull your hands to your sides, pinching your shoulders together. Keep a relaxed but firm grip on the band. Your back should remain upright and your legs straight. You should feel the effort in your back, shoulders and biceps.

Hold for one second. Slowly return your hands to the starting position. Perform eight to twelve repetitions.

Weight room equivalent: Seated or compound row

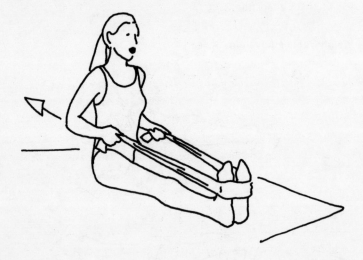

Lateral Raise

Works the deltoid and rotator cuff muscles in the shoulders.

Standing with your arms at your sides and your feet shoulder-width apart, hold a dumbbell in each hand.

Keeping your arms straight and your palms facing in, lift your hands to the side to shoulder height. Keep your elbows slightly bent. You should feel the effort in your shoulders, not your neck or jaw.

Hold for one second, then slowly lower your arms back to your sides. Perform eight to twelve repetitions.

Variation: You can also do this exercise with an exercise band looped around each foot.

Weight room equivalent: Lateral raise machine

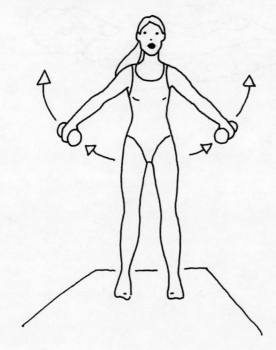

Back Extension

Targets your lower back muscles.

Lie face down on the floor with your hands at your sides, next to your hips. Slowly raise your shoulders and chest off the floor about twelve centimetres/five inches by contracting your back muscles. Keep your lower body relaxed and your head in line with your upper body.

Hold for one second, then slowly lower your upper body to within one inch of the floor.

Perform eight to twelve repetitions.

Weight room equivalent: Lower back machine

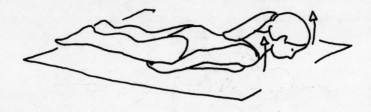

Crunch

Works all your abdominal muscles.

Lie on the floor on your back with your knees bent at a 90-degree angle. Your feet should be flat on the floor. Cross your arms across your chest.

Slowly contract your abdominal muscles and raise your shoulder blades off the floor. Keep your head in line with your body – your chin off your chest, your neck relaxed. (Tip: keep your eyes focused on your knees.)

Briefly hold this position, then slowly lower yourself back down to the floor. Do as many repetitions as you can while maintaining good form.

Weight room equivalent: Abdominal machine

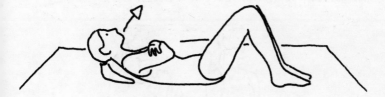

Arm Curl

Targets your biceps.

Stand upright with your arms at your sides, your feet about shoulder-width apart and your knees slightly bent.

Grasp one end of the exercise band with your right hand, palm facing forward, and place your right foot on the other end. There should be a slight tension in the band.

Slowly bend your arm and bring your hand to your shoulder, keeping your elbow still and your back straight.

Hold for one second, then slowly return to the starting position. Do eight to twelve repetitions, then repeat on your left side.

Variation: You can also do this exercise using a dumbbell instead of the exercise band.

Weight room equivalent: Arm curl or biceps curl

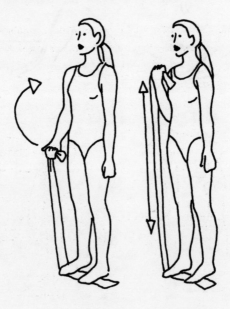

Rear Extension

Works your triceps.

Stand to the right of a weight bench or behind a chair. Bend forward at the waist and place your left hand on the chair or bench. If you're using a bench, you can place your left knee on the bench for support.

Hold the dumbbell in your right hand, with your right elbow bent to a 90-degree angle and your upper arm next to your torso, parallel to the floor. Keep your palm facing in and the weight close to your side.

Straighten your arm in back of you to lift the weight, keeping your elbow and upper arm still. Don't twist your back or lock your elbow.

When your arm is straight behind you and parallel to the floor, pause for one second. Return to the starting position. Perform eight to twelve repetitions, then switch arms and repeat on the opposite side.

Variation: You can perform this exercise with a resistance band by stepping on one end with your foot and holding the other end in your hand.

Weight room equivalent: Triceps extension

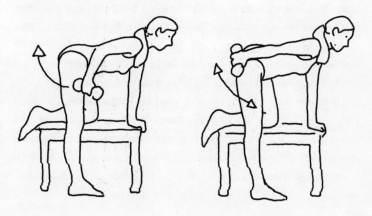

Getting Your Doctor's Okay to Exercise

If you're just beginning an exercise programme, show this plan to your doctor to make sure it's appropriate for you. If you have any of the following health conditions, you may need to be on a modified exercise programme under your doctor's supervision:

- Heart disease or other heart condition
- High blood pressure
- Pregnancy
- History of breathing problems (including asthma)
- Chest pain during physical activity
- Bone or joint problems
- Diabetes
- Previous episodes of dizziness or loss of consciousness

Your Weekly Exercise Plan

If you're new to exercise, you'll need to ease into your exercise routine – building up from a 15 minute to an hour's walk during your first few weeks, for example. This plan will help you build up your stamina while minimizing your risk of injury during the first six weeks. Each week, you'll increase and extend your activities until you're going full force during the sixth week and beyond.

If at any time you find you've increased your intensity beyond your fitness level, go back to your previous fitness routine until you feel it has become too easy. Then you can move on to the next week on the plan. By the same token, if week one feels too easy for your fitness level, skip ahead to a week where you feel comfortable. Remember: if you don't feel like you're working hard enough, you should be increasing the intensity or duration of your activity. For strength training, you should be using a heavier weight or increasing the number of sets.

As you'll see, the plan gives you one day off a week. You can take this day whenever you choose – perhaps on a particularly hectic day when you just can't squeeze in a workout.

All you need to do now is choose the aerobic activity you've decided to try, make a list of the equipment and clothing you'll need, and get moving! (Of course, don't forget to get your doctor's go-ahead before you begin.)

WEEK ONE

SUNDAY
Warm-up 5 minutes
Stretch 5 minutes
Aerobic Activity 15–20 minutes
Stretch 5 minutes

MONDAY
Warm-up 5 minutes
Stretch 5 minutes
Strength Training Routine: 1 set
    of all exercises (8–12 reps)
Stretch 5 minutes

TUESDAY
Warm-up 5 minutes
Stretch 5 minutes
Aerobic Activity 15–20 minutes
Stretch 5 minutes

WEDNESDAY
Day Off

THURSDAY
Warm-up 5 minutes
Stretch 5 minutes
Strength Training Routine: 1 set
    of all exercises (8–12 reps)
Stretch 5 minutes

FRIDAY
Warm-up 5 minutes
Stretch 5 minutes
Aerobic Activity 15–20 minutes
Stretch 5 minutes

SATURDAY
Fun Day*

*Fun Days can be taken on any day of the week, although weekends are usually most convenient. Use this as an occasion to be active with your family or friends. Go for a long walk, try ice-skating at your local sports centre, take a trip to the beach and swim or walk along coastline. Maybe you and your partner always wanted to try horseriding or take tae kwon do. Seize the day!

WEEK TWO

SUNDAY

Warm-up 5 minutes

Stretch 5 minutes

Aerobic Activity 25 minutes

Stretch 5 minutes

MONDAY

Warm-up 5 minutes

Stretch 5 minutes

Strength Training Routine: 1 set
    of all exercises (12–15 reps)

Stretch 5 minutes

TUESDAY

Warm-up 5 minutes

Stretch 5 minutes

Aerobic Activity 25 minutes

Stretch 5 minutes

WEDNESDAY

Warm-up 5 minutes

Stretch 5 minutes

Strength Training Routine: 1 set
    of all exercises (12–15 reps)

Stretch 5 minutes

THURSDAY

Day off

FRIDAY

Warm-up 5 minutes

Stretch 5 minutes

Aerobic Activity 25 minutes

Stretch 5 minutes

SATURDAY

Fun Day*

WEEK THREE

SUNDAY
Warm-up 5 minutes
Stretch 5 minutes
Aerobic Activity 30–35 minutes
Cool-down & Stretch 10 minutes

MONDAY
Day Off

TUESDAY
Warm-up 5 minutes
Stretch 5 minutes
Aerobic Activity 30–35 minutes
Cool-down & Stretch 10 minutes

WEDNESDAY
Warm-up 5 minutes
Stretch 5 minutes
Strength Training Routine: 2 sets
    of all exercises (8 reps)
Stretch 5 minutes

THURSDAY
Warm-up 5 minutes
Stretch 5 minutes
Aerobic Activity 40 minutes
Cool-down & Stretch 10 minutes

FRIDAY
Warm-up 5 minutes
Stretch 5 minutes
Strength Training Routine: 2 sets
    of all exercises (8 reps)
Stretch 5 minutes

SATURDAY
Fun Day*

WEEK FOUR

SUNDAY
Warm-up 5 minutes
Stretch 5 minutes
Aerobic Activity 40 minutes
Cool-down & Stretch 10 minutes

MONDAY
Warm-up 5 minutes
Stretch 5 minutes
Strength Training Routine: 2 sets
    of all exercises (12 reps)
Aerobic Activity 20 minutes
Cool-down & Stretch 10 minutes

TUESDAY
Warm-up 5 minutes
Stretch 5 minutes
Aerobic Activity 40 minutes
Cool-down & Stretch 10 minutes

WEDNESDAY
Day Off

THURSDAY
Warm-up 5 minutes
Stretch 5 minutes
Aerobic Activity 45–50 minutes
Cool-down & Stretch 10 minutes

FRIDAY
Warm-up 5 minutes
Stretch 5 minutes
Strength Training Routine: 2 sets
    of all exercises (12 reps)
Aerobic Activity 20 minutes
Cool-down & Stretch 10 minutes

SATURDAY
Fun Day*

WEEK FIVE

SUNDAY
Warm-up 5 minutes
Stretch 5 minutes
Aerobic Activity 45–50 minutes
Cool-down & Stretch 10 minutes

MONDAY
Warm-up 5 minutes
Stretch 5 minutes
Strength Training Routine: 2 sets
    of all exercises (15 reps)
Aerobic Activity 25 minutes
Cool-down & Stretch 10 minutes

TUESDAY
Warm-up 5 minutes
Stretch 5 minutes
Aerobic Activity 45–50 minutes
Cool-down & Stretch 10 minutes

WEDNESDAY
Warm-up 5 minutes
Stretch 5 minutes
Strength Training Routine: 2 sets
    of all exercises (15 reps)
Aerobic Activity 25 minutes
Cool-down & Stretch 10 minutes

THURSDAY
Warm-up 5 minutes
Aerobic Activity 30 minutes
Cool-down & Stretch 10 minutes
Stretch 5 minutes
Strength Training Routine: 1 set
    (8 reps) at heavier weight and
    1 set (12 reps) at regular
    weight

FRIDAY
Day Off

SATURDAY
Fun Day*

WEEK SIX

SUNDAY
Day Off

MONDAY
Warm-up 5 minutes
Stretch 5 minutes
Aerobic Activity 50 minutes–
    1 hour
Cool-down & Stretch 10 minutes

TUESDAY
Warm-up 5 minutes
Stretch 5 minutes
Aerobic Activity 30 minutes
Cool-down & Stretch 10 minutes
Strength Training Routine: 1 set
    (8 reps) at heavier weight and
    1 set (12 reps) at regular
    weight

WEDNESDAY
Warm-up 5 minutes
Stretch 5 minutes
Aerobic Activity 50 minutes–
    1 hour
Cool-down & Stretch 10 minutes

THURSDAY
Warm-up 5 minutes
Aerobic Activity 30 minutes
Stretch 5 minutes
Strength Training Routine: 1 set
    (8 reps) at heavier weight and
    1 set (12 reps) at regular
    weight
Cool-down & Stretch 10 minutes

FRIDAY
Warm-up 5 minutes
Stretch 5 minutes
Aerobic Activity 50 minutes–
    1 hour
Cool Down & Stretch 10 minutes

SATURDAY
Fun Day*

You're off to a great start!
Remember: it's important to
choose exercises you enjoy doing.
If you get bored, then you'll know
it's time to vary your workouts, or
look for a new activity altogether.
Your body doesn't care how you
get it moving, as long as you're
working your heart and the rest of
your muscles. Keep it up, and
revel in the way you feel!

Creating Your Personal Relaxation Plan

How many times have you used food to take the edge off a particularly trying day? When you have a hard time at work, it's easy enough – *too easy* – to lose yourself in a desk-drawer stash of chocolate biscuits. After you've run twenty minutes late for every errand and appointment you had all day, crashing out in front of the TV with a selection of your favourite snacks can be an irresistible way to forget all the stress. But this quick-fix relief comes with a hefty price tag – unwanted pounds.

Exercise can be a great stress reliever, but it's all about *invigoration;* ideally, it should be offset with an equally important dose of *relaxation.* The Slim•Fast Makeover is designed to help you achieve that relaxation, giving you a kind of mini-holiday every single day – a small pocket of time to clear your mind and step away from the daily stresses of life.

Relaxation doesn't mean sinking into your sofa and vegging out in front of the TV – a time when you may be doing nothing, but your mind may well be worrying over the stresses of the day. True relaxation is the art of *letting go.* It's all about releasing tension from your muscles and sweeping away troubling thoughts. And in order to achieve complete relaxation, both mind and body must be free of that tension.

Bad Habits – And How to Ban Them

It's one of life's great lessons: we are our own caretakers – or, to put it another way, we're our own mothers. If we don't take care of ourselves, it won't get done. No one can be a good parent if they spend all their time making excuses, saying 'Oh, I'm too busy working,' or

'I can't take care of you – I've got friends who need me.' Likewise, if you want to lead a happy life, the best thing you can do is stop making excuses and start turning your attention to taking care of yourself.

Here's one thing I've learned about myself: whenever I catch myself falling into a little self-destructive pattern – taking on everyone else's problems as my own – I feel like going straight to the refrigerator for a dose of comfort food. I used to be the same way about smoking. Before I quit, whenever I was taking on too much stress I'd reach for a cigarette; sometimes I'd have a cigarette in one hand and a lit match in the other before I realized what I was doing.

I've banished my old stress-binge eating habits just the same way I quit smoking: every time I got one of those anxious 'hunger' pangs, I'd take a deep breath and remove myself from the situation to focus on exactly what I was feeling. Usually it only takes five or ten minutes of concentration before your equilibrium settles back into place. And so what if you feel like crying or kicking something? Everyone feels that way every now and then; if you're not alone, head for the bathroom or take a walk around the block. It's a nice way to sneak a little private time into your own life. Try making this a practice, and if you can do it for twenty-one days, the way I did, you'll find you've kicked the bad-eating habit.

Good Habits – And How to Make Them

We are creatures of habit, but what many people never realize is that we can choose our habits. Just as we owe it to ourselves to drop our bad habits, it's in our best interest to cultivate the positive habits that make up a healthy lifestyle.

Here's one: *breathe.* The most important thing we do in life is breathing, but most of us never give it a second thought. Air is our number one food; it comes before water, before eatables, before anything. I make it a point to take deep breaths all day long, because the body runs on oxygen – the oxygen we draw from the air into our lungs, which then enriches the blood and fuels the rest of our bodily functions. Exercise will help you breathe deeply, but even when you're just sitting at your desk quietly, every so often pull in a nice, long breath of air. It'll do you good.

Here's another: *drink water.* Most of us don't get as much as we need. I keep water bottles with me wherever I go: by my desk, in the car, by the TV – in every room in the house, in fact. Since I started upping my water intake (I make it a point to have at least six big glasses a day, always trying for eight), I find that everything works better – especially my plumbing. And here's another discovery I made: it works wonders for wrinkles! It turns out moisturizing from the inside is even more important than applying oils or creams on the outside.

The all-important third habit: *eat right.* Slim•Fast makes it easy with two shakes a day, but they didn't come up with the phrase 'sensible dinner' for nothing. It's important to eat as many fresh foods, and as few processed foods, as possible. Reduce your intake of heavy meats and increase your vegetables and fruits to compensate. It's much easier to find a wide range of organic foods than it used to be, and many more people every year are introducing tofu and other soya dishes into their diets. I also make it a point to cook with olive oil, which is the healthiest variety and to have good raw vegetables on hand for snacking all day long.

And, personally, I do believe in taking *vitamins and minerals* every day. Every morning, along with my Slim•Fast, I take vitamin C and beta-carotene; at lunch I take vitamin E and selenium, along with a calcium-magnesium combination and one aspirin (because my family has a history of heart disease). There are a lot of other supplements on the market, of course, and there seem to be more cropping up all the time. But these are my staples, the ones I've been taking every day for years.

Eliciting the Relaxation Response

To 'make over' your mind and mental outlook, the plan will teach you how to elicit 'the relaxation response' – a term coined by relaxation researcher Herbert Benson, M.D., author of *Timeless Healing*. You'll actually be calming all your body's systems. You'll lower your blood pressure and decrease your heart rate and breathing rate. Research also suggests that eliciting the relaxation response boosts your brain's production of the feel-good chemicals serotonin and endorphins, which will increase your sense of calm and happiness.

In over two decades of research, Benson and his colleagues have determined that getting your body into a relaxed state can have a host of health benefits, from lowering your risk of heart disease to curing insomnia to restoring a happier outlook to your life. Eliciting the relaxation response has another added benefit: it can actually help reduce your craving for sweets by regulating the release of cortisol, a stress hormone that can wreak havoc with blood sugar levels and convince your body it needs more sugar.

Given all these obvious advantages, it's important to learn to relax on demand – even if it means actively ignoring the source of your stress. Choose one of the relaxation techniques below (or try a different technique each day); *give yourself fifteen to twenty minutes a day to get your body into a completely relaxed state.* Skip that mediocre sitcom or close your door during your coffee break at work. Just be sure to choose a time of day when you can unplug the phone and be free of any distractions.

Your Getaway Options

The traditional way Dr Benson has developed and tested this method of eliciting the relaxation response: first, sit comfortably and pick a focus word or short phrase that's meaningful to you. Close your eyes and relax your muscles. Now, breathe slowly and naturally, repeating your focus word or phrase silently as you exhale.

Throughout, assume a passive attitude. Don't worry about whether you're performing the technique correctly. When other thoughts come to mind, simply let them pass without pondering them. Gently return to your repetition. Continue for fifteen to twenty minutes. You may open your eyes to check the time, but don't use an alarm – it'll only disrupt your relaxation. When you finish, sit quietly for a minute or so, at first with your eyes closed and then with your eyes open. Remain seated for one or two minutes before standing.

Progressive muscle relaxation Sit in a comfortable chair with back and head support, or lie on a lightly cushioned mat on the floor. (A bed is too soft and will make you more likely to fall asleep.) Tense each of your muscles one at a time; inhale and slowly exhale as you release the tension from your muscles. Begin with your face by wrinkling your forehead and shutting your eyes as tight as you can. Exhale and release. Then tense your neck and shoulders by drawing your shoulders up into a shrug. Exhale and release. Work your way down to your arms and hands, pressing your palms together with your elbows pointing outward and push as hard as you can. Exhale and release. Contract your stomach. Exhale and release. Arch your back and release. Now tense your hips and buttocks, pressing your legs and heels against the surface beneath you. Exhale and release. Point and flex your toes and release.

Now tense all your muscles at once. Then take a deep breath, hold it, then exhale slowly as you relax the muscles, letting go of the tension. Feel your body at rest and enjoy this state of relaxation for several minutes. When you're first learning this technique, you may want to create a tape recording, reading slowly through the above instructions. You can play the recording while you're relaxing your muscles to make sure you don't skip any of the muscle groups.

Meditation The focused awareness that comes with meditation can let you appreciate the interconnectedness of all living things. Sit comfortably in an upright position with your head, neck and back erect but not stiff. You can sit in a straight-backed chair or cross-legged on the floor. Choose a single object of focus like your breathing or the light of a candle. Concentrate on the qualities of that object – the sounds, sensations, or appearance – as they enter into your awareness.

You can also practice meditation in a natural setting such as a garden, or while sitting by a window. Watch the sun set, the clouds drift, or the stars twinkle, and focus on the air flowing in and out of your body as you breathe. Appreciating the beauty of nature allows you to transcend your own problems and reminds you of how vast the world really is.

Strike a pose Yoga can help increase your sense of serenity. What's more, you'll be improving your body tone and flexibility at the same time. You should move through the various poses slowly and mindfully to get the benefit of relaxation. You can learn yoga by taking a class (which is probably the best method, since an instructor can correct your form) or through a book or video.

Relaxation quickie When you feel your tension rising, you may not be in a position to take a twenty-minute relaxation break. In these situations, you can use this quick and effective technique described by Dr Christian Northrup. Press your hand over your heart and close your eyes. While breathing deeply, recall someone or something you love completely and unconditionally. Feel that loving feeling for a minute or so. Open your eyes and take a deep breath. It'll help you remember what life is really all about.

Now that you've got the basics of the Slim•Fast Makeover, you're ready to put it all together and begin living a new life. At times, you'll find you need to work hard to maintain your healthy habits. Just remember how good you feel and how great you've already begun to look as a result of your new life. Reward yourself once in a while with a new outfit or a night out on the town. In fact, that's what the next chapter is all about – celebrating your new life. You'll see that you can still eat out and enjoy parties while maintaining your healthy lifestyle. It's time to have your cake and eat it, too!

8

celebrate your new life!

As you plan and plot your meals, track your exercise and pencil in your relaxation efforts, remember one of the most important elements of the Slim•Fast Makeover: having fun. Fun is often the forgotten factor. After all, on most diets you deprive yourself until you reach your ultimate weight-loss goal – and then you're so hard up for fun that you can hardly be blamed for going overboard to make up for all those weeks of deprivation.

The Slim•Fast Makeover is all about getting pleasure in your life. The Slim•Fast products taste like milk shakes and chocolate bars for one reason: so you'll enjoy them. Eating should always be a pleasurable experience. You may be controlling the amount of food you put in your mouth, but you should still be able to savour every mouthful. By the same token, your fitness activities should be fun and leave you feeling invigorated. Your relaxation practices should help you tap into the joy that comes with being alive and experiencing the simple pleasures of the world around you.

So if you've gotten this far into the plan, your life should already have become more enjoyable, filled with good food, invigorating exercise and the excitement that comes from improving your life. Still, you may be wondering about some aspects of everyday life that might seem hard to reconcile with all your plans. What about my favourite restaurants? What about the office Christmas party? How will I make it through my family reunion without over indulging?

But there's no need to worry. You can live your normal social life without worrying about sacrificing your weight-loss efforts. All you need are some strategies for dealing with these situations.

You can eat out at good restaurants and live through a brush with a party buffet, as long as you make smart selections. Just think before you read. You can even eat a little fast food occasionally. The key is moderation. Just use common sense – restrict your dining-out plans to once a week instead of picking up takeaway two or three nights a week. Give yourself the green light to do anything you really want to do, but know when to flash the red light – stop before you feel too full. If you'll take the time to develop sensible strategies for navigating those tempting pitfalls, you'll have the satisfaction of making your own decisions about what goes into your body and how you feel every week.

Celebrating your new life also means finding pleasure in so much more than just food. For many of us food is a main source of pleasure, and that's fine – but it shouldn't be the *principal* source of comfort or solace. With your new body and new life, you'll find other outlets for pleasure and fun. Need to get some new clothes to fit your new body size? Be a little carefree and pick up a high-fashion shirt you normally wouldn't buy or a pair of trousers in the latest colour. Try a different hairstyle to go with your new body and your new attitude. As part of your transformation, you may even find yourself feeling sexier; after all, your sex drive is a barometer of your overall health, and being in shape can make things easier in the bedroom on any number of levels – from physical stamina to confidence. Not a bad bonus, right?

Here are a few smart strategies to keep in mind as you venture out in the world.

Smart Strategy 1: Map Out a Plan When Going to a Restaurant

Eating out *can* throw a wrench into your weight-loss efforts, if you're not careful about what you put in your mouth. Still, there's no reason to forsake this pleasure for the good of your waistline. Eat out once or twice a week at most, and follow these rules to navigate the minefield of temptations:

Analyse your own eating personality If you tend to go overboard when you go to a restaurant famished, try eating a light snack beforehand. A Slim•Fast snack bar or a piece of fruit with a small piece of cheese should keep hunger at bay, so you won't be as tempted to eat three rolls before your starter. On the other hand, if you know you can't restrict yourself when eating out, stick with much lighter meals earlier in the day. (If you have a Slim•Fast shake for both breakfast and lunch, you should feel just right for a healthy dinner.)

Beware of the bread basket Tell your waiter not to bring any bread to the table if the sight or scent of it is too tempting. If you still can't resist, take one piece (without butter) and divide it into three parts. Eat the first before you order, the second while waiting for the meal and the third with your meal (with luck you won't even be tempted by then). This kind of portion control is a good strategy for any eating situation.

Order from the starter or salad sections of the menu Treating a starter as a main course is a good way to save on calories, since they come in smaller portions. A soup and side salad can also make a filling meal, without the added calories and fat. But beware, salads also come huge enough to feed two people. A plate filled with plain fresh vegetables won't contain many calories – but add some dressing, avocado, cheese, fish, or chicken to the mix and you've got a calorie-packed meal. If there's a huge salad you're dying to have, split it with your dining partner or ask for a side-salad portion.

Dine à la carte You may be inclined to order a full meal – starter, dessert, and all – if it costs less than the sum of its parts. But this plan only sets you up to eat more. Don't force down a dessert just because it's included – especially if you aren't really hungry.

Get the dressing on the side Many salads are smothered in high-fat dressing and can end up being as fattening as a huge steak. Ask the waiter how the salad is dressed and if you can have the dressing served separately so that you can drizzle it over yourself.

Watch for hidden calories Many meals are loaded with calories, added in subtle ways. Oils are often added to tomato sauces; rich gravies or cream sauces are poured over meats and vegetables. A low-fat fillet of fish can be turned into a vehicle for fat by being breaded and fried. In general, the plainer the food, the better. Anything grilled, with a light sprinkling of spices, tends to be lower in calories than something bathed in a thicker sauce.

Mind the alcohol Alcohol is loaded with calories, and it's easy to consume more than you want while you're in the social spirit. Stick to one glass of wine or beer with dinner, or a dessert aperitif. Remember, a small beer or glass of wine contains about 100 calories.

Make dessert conditional Before you order dessert, ask yourself if you're really still hungry and if the dessert is within your calorie budget for the day. Try some low-calorie, healthy dessert options such as fresh raspberries sprinkled on a small scoop of sorbet, or strawberries topped with a tiny squirt of whipped cream.

Engage your partner Try to eat out with someone who will help you keep your temptations in check. The two of you can decide in advance what to order, before your restraint is weakened. Your partner can keep the breadbasket in a safe place, and refrain from pushing drinks or dessert.

Let yourself off the hook If you eat more than you planned, don't consider it a catastrophe. Remember, it's unrealistic to think you'll never overeat. What you don't want to do is quit your weight-loss efforts because you think you've blown it. Keep the event in perspective and resolve to make a better go of it next time.

Smart Strategy 2: With Fast Food, Think Salads and Child-Size Portions

You don't necessarily need to avoid fast-food establishments altogether. By popular demand, fast-food restaurants have evolved to include some healthier options. Their chicken dishes can be lower in fat and calories than beef dishes – as long as you choose grilled dishes instead of fried chicken or nuggets. Healthier oils are being used to cook French fries in some places, though they're still loaded with the same amount of fat and calories. If you choose selectively, it is possible to walk into a fast-food restaurant and escape with a reasonable meal.

Stay away from the breaded and fried Anything that's covered in batter, grease, or a thick sauce is bound to be loaded with fat and calories. Healthy low-fat options include a skinless grilled chicken breast sandwich topped with chopped vegetables, a plain grilled fish, or a grilled vegetable burger. Try a plain baked potato or rice instead of fries.

Stick with child-size portions If you must order fries, get the small size. If you have a hankering for a hamburger, order a child-size meal. Reducing portion sizes will help keep calories and fat under control.

Forgo regular soft drinks Go for diet drinks rather than regular versions, which are loaded with sugar and empty calories. And stay away from milkshakes, which can have more calories and fat than your main course.

Smart Strategy 3: Party! (with Restraint)

Parties can be major pitfalls when you're trying to lose weight, since you have no control over what is served. Even the seemingly harmless handfuls of nibbles you grab here and there from tables can really add up. Still, you don't need to skip parties altogether. Just go with a game plan like this one.

Don't arrive hungry Take the edge off hunger before you leave home by eating something light but satisfying, like a few crackers with some low-fat spread or a Slim•Fast snack bar.

Allow yourself a little splurge Denying yourself all the temptations you see at parties could set you up for an eating binge when you get home. When you first arrive, survey the scene and see which food looks the most tempting. Allow yourself that piece of chocolate fudge or slice of cheesecake, but don't try everything. If you want to sample a few things, stick with modest portions and smaller bites. You'll satisfy your curiosity without packing in the calories.

Avoid mindless eating This is hard to do at a party when you're chattering away and not really paying attention to what you're putting in your mouth. Rather than eating throughout the party, do one modest round of the finger foods and one of the desserts and avoid going back for seconds.

Keep in mind that alcohol's calories count Having two or three drinks at a party can send your daily calorie count spinning out of control. If you're going to indulge in alcohol, stick with lower-calorie foods. Better yet, have just one drink and then stick with a low-calorie option.

Smart Strategy 4: Use a Lapse to Help Get You Back on Track

In the name of having a little fun, you may find you want to let the rules slide from time to time. Perhaps you used your two-week holiday as a break from your makeover plan. Or maybe you've been cheating a little more each day. The fact is, everyone cheats from time to time – including people who are successful at maintaining a weight loss. The key is in how you deal with these lapses – whether you throw in the towel or get yourself back on track. Once you realize you've fallen off the wagon, follow these seven steps developed by psychologist G. Alan Marlatt, Ph.D.

Step 1: Stop, look and listen A lapse is a signal of impending danger, like flashing lights at a railway crossing. Stop a moment – especially if the lapse is still in progress – and examine the situation. Can you afford this lapse? Consider removing yourself to a safe situation away from the temptations to avoid overindulging.

Step 2: Stay calm If you get anxious or blame yourself for the lapse, you may conclude that you're a hopeless binge eater with no control. Try to separate yourself from the situation and realize what an objective observer would – that one lapse doesn't make your efforts a failure.

Step 3: Renew your weight-loss vows Take a minute to remind yourself of how far you've come and how sad it would be if one lapse cancelled out all your work. Remind yourself of your goals and renew the vows you made when you began the programme.

Step 4: Analyse the lapse situation Instead of blaming yourself for letting go, use the situation to learn what places you at risk. Do certain feelings trigger overeating? Does the presence of food or other activities tempt you consistently? Have you done anything to defend against the urge? Did it work? Why or why not? What would you do differently in the future?

Step 5: Take charge immediately Leap into action; waiting is just another excuse for letting go. Leave the house, throw the remaining food out, or do whatever works for you. You might try to schedule a workout and plan your next day's meals to get yourself back on track.

Step 6: Make Slim•Fast your next meal This can be a great way to get back on track.

Step 7: Ask for help Partners, friends, co-workers and others can be a real source of support, providing perspective and offering the encouragement you may need.

Smart Strategy 5: Live Your Life with Style

Style has nothing to do with body size, and it isn't about settling for clothes that 'just fit' either. Your personal style should feature clothes that fit your life and flatter your body. If you're trying to lose weight – whether it's 4 kilograms or 24 – you'll certainly need to consider your changing body in the choices you make. You also need to consider the type of life you lead: whether you work in a corporate or a casual environment, what you do in your spare time and so on. On top of this, you should consider your own personal style preferences (are you classic or trendy? quiet or outgoing?) and taste in colour. When all of these things come together, your own individual style begins to emerge. This style will reflect the new you that you've become.

Thankfully, designers and manufacturers have finally started to realize that the majority of women are not size 10–12 and that shapeless tent dresses just won't do anymore for large-size women. These women want the four Fs: fit, function and figure-flattery. Clothes that provide ample coverage while streamlining your shape can do wonders for your self-confidence while you're trying to lose weight. Finding clothes that move smoothly from one point on the scale to the next – as well as from day to night and season to season – can help you maintain your sense of style and feel good about the way you look.

Highlight what you like and minimize what you don't You want to bring out your body's best features. Long sleeves can cover fuller arms, while a well-cut blouse flatters a large bust and emphasizes shoulders. If you've got a large bottom, wear an A-line or flared skirt (not pleated or form-fitting) and loose-fitting trousers.

Shop before you drop Don't wait until you get to your goal weight before buying new clothes. Purchasing a great-where-you-are wardrobe basic, like a classic shirt, tells you that you deserve to look good now, though you can still wear it as you lose weight. Also, the better you feel about yourself in clothes, the more motivated you'll be to move into a smaller size.

Stay in touch with your body Knowing your good and not-so-good points will help you dress for slimming success. Follow this colour adage: dark recedes and light reflects. Dark colours should stay below the hips, light colours above. To maximize height and slenderness, wear all one colour. You should also take note of where you gain and lose weight first. When choosing an outfit, give yourself a little extra room in these areas to allow for a 1–1.5kg (2–3lb) weight fluctuation.

Try a body shaper If you're working out hard, but not getting the results as quickly as you'd like, you can still flatten your stomach and smooth out your hips with the new body shapers. Updated and more comfortable versions of the traditional girdle, they're made from body-sleeking Spandex and can be found in most women's lingerie departments.

Avoid fattening styles While there are many clothes styles that can flatter, there are also quite a few that should be avoided: big floral patterns; bold prints; big patch pockets; oversize buttons, touches and trims; horizontal patterns; trousers with turn-ups; bulky fabrics; big wide belts; and head-hugging hats.

What's most important is that you find the time to enjoy yourself and break free from the daily grind. Socializing with friends and having fun with your family can renew your spirit and give you a fresh outlook on life. The thing to keep in mind is, living healthy and having fun don't need to be mutually exclusive. Both are essential to the success of your makeover plan.

9

maintaining your makeover

If you've given yourself the Slim•Fast Makeover, you've given yourself a great gift. You've improved your health and weight. You've improved the physical fitness of your body and the spiritual fitness of your mind. You've taken charge of your life to make each day more fulfilling than the day before. As you continue in the coming weeks and months, you're in the perfect position to transform your life for good.

This book may be coming to an end, but your makeover is just beginning. As you'll see, it will continue to evolve as you lose weight and gain the energy to do things you never thought possible. You'll probably want to try new fitness activities, to travel to new places, to update your look and your wardrobe. You'll crave excitement from your life, and start looking for new adventures. If you allow this sense of freshness and excitement to refresh you every day, you should have no trouble staying on the makeover plan.

If you've been concerned about improving your health, the makeover will continue to help. Maintaining a healthy weight can help prevent many of the diseases associated with the ageing process. You'll have a lower risk of developing heart disease, diabetes and certain cancers. The combination of exercising and eating a nutritious, calcium-rich, well-balanced diet that includes Slim•Fast can help stave off osteoporosis and keep your immune system finely tuned. Your body will thank you, and you'll continue to feel and look better than you ever have in your life.

At some point along the way, you should reach a weight you're happy with and feel satisfied with your fitness level. You'll probably think to yourself, 'I feel good staying just where I am.' It's at this point that you may be tempted to revert back to your old ways; after all, we live in a goal-oriented society and we're used to putting forth effort just long enough to receive our rewards.

If you find yourself slipping back into your old habits, think about how you've been feeling lately. Do you have less energy? Are you feeling bloated and out of sorts? Are your trousers feeling tighter? Remember the point of the Slim●Fast Makeover: to infuse you with good health, energy and vitality. If you abandon the makeover, your body will let you know. You'll also find your weight creeping back up the scale. The truth is, unless you follow the healthy principles you've learned, it won't take long for your body to revert to its old shape.

Remember, in order to maintain a weight loss, you need to eat far fewer calories than you ate at your old weight. The best way to do this is to follow the nutrition plan and replace one meal a day with a Slim●Fast product – especially if you find yourself gaining weight. Don't allow yourself to get into a meal rut (if it's Tuesday, it must be salmon). Use the dozens of recipes throughout this book to vary your cooking and keep your taste buds tantalized. And make an effort to try new fruits and vegetables that catch your eye in the supermarket. The best way to stick with any plan, after all, is to keep it interesting.

You should also take measures to avoid boredom with your fitness programme. The minute you feel you're no longer being challenged, increase the intensity or duration of your workouts, or switch to a new activity altogether. If you've pedaled too many miles on the stationary bike or climbed too many stairs on the stair machine, try taking a step or kick-boxing class. If you've worn down the path that takes you around your neighbourhood, find a new walking route that challenges you with hills. The more you can make over your makeover as you go, the better off you'll be.

You may even find that you need to revamp your relaxation plan from time to time. You should feel invigorated, not bored, after practising your technique. Feel free to try a new technique if you find your old one is putting you to sleep rather than relaxing you.

As you can see, the Slim•Fast Makeover has fail-safes that should keep you from getting bored with the plan. There are so many eating, exercise and relaxation options here that you can re-create your plan every couple of weeks. The key is to try out new options once you find that you're getting stuck in a rut.

To gauge how you're doing on your makeover, you need to continue to fill in your makeover diary *every day*. Read through your diary every week to get a quick assessment of how you feel on the plan. At the beginning of each week, think about what is or isn't working for you, and then implement new options to keep your plan fresh.

At certain times you'll probably be more faithful to the makeover plan than at others. Don't beat yourself up or sit in judgment of yourself if you cheat a little! Just remember how great you feel when you're sticking with your plan and use that as a motivation to get back on track. Feeling guilty is self-defeating and can actually cause you to lose faith. Whatever you do, never let yourself think 'Oh, what the heck – I've already blown it.' It ain't over till it's over – till you have the life you want.

As the saying goes, *Today is the first day of the rest of your life.* Make today the day you begin anew – whether you're beginning your makeover for the first time or renewing your commitment to the plan. Here's to you and your new life!

Lauren Hutton

index